Praise for *Yoga Nidra Meditations*

"Julie is a master at helping us relax. In her new book she offers her own relaxation scripts, as well as a sampling from other gifted teachers, that guide us in the essentials of relaxation for different states of body and mind. This book is one to keep on the bedside and buy a couple for stressed out friends, they will thank you."

—Nischala Joy Devi, author of *The Secret Power of Yoga*, *The Namaste Effect,* and *The Healing Path of Yoga*

"This beautifully written book is well-laid out, easy to follow, and chock full of helpful and powerful information. The relaxation scripts are incredible and are sure to assist in helping everyone to find more peace, ease, and healing in their lives. This is a much-needed guide in times of discomfort and stress."

—M. Mala Cunningham, PhD, C-IAYT, counseling psychologist, university faculty, and specialist in medical yoga, neuroscience, and mindfulness

"Julie Lusk's inspirational book provides an indispensable guide to the healing practice of Yoga Nidra … Julie's expertise and generous heart shine through and make her the perfect companion to guide you along the Yoga Nidra path. This is a book to be treasured and returned to over again."

—Jilly Shipway, author of *Yoga Through the Year* and *Yoga by the Stars*

"Having experienced several of the Yoga Nidra practices from this book, taught by Julie herself, I can confidently say that they are immensely enjoyable and relaxing. Each practice guides you in a unique way, but all of them leave you with a profound sense of well-being."

—Zac Parker, MA, RYT-500, online programs coordinator at Yogaville

"Julie Lusk has captured the essence of Yoga Nidra, meditation, and beyond from the great masters, present and past, and has added her own great contributions. Highly recommended."

—Larry Payne, PhD E-RYT500, author of *AARP's Yoga Af*

"Julie Lusk created this work in the spirit of Yoga Nidra—with relaxed expectation of divine blessings—and she effortlessly transmits that peaceful joy through these healing scripts … Julie brings together an inspired crew with centuries of combined experience to make this path of deep healing available in our daily lives."

—Judith Boice, award-winning author of *The Green Medicine Chest* and practicing naturopathic physician

"Julie Lusk's clear, direct, joyful voice explains everything you ever wanted to know about Yoga Nidra. Whether you are a novice or an experienced practitioner, this is your go-to reference book, explaining how, where, and when to practice it, the philosophy behind it, ways to get the most out of it, tips for instructing others, and a whole cache of scripts … her sheer delight with this practice shines through every joyful page."

—Belleruth Naparstek, ACSW, BCD, author of *Invisible Heroes* and producer of the Health Journeys Guided Imagery and Meditation audio library

"Master yoga teacher Julie Lusk has enthusiastically and lovingly taken the ancient subject of Yoga Nidra and made it useful and relevant for today. The meditations are clear, practical, and uplifting. It truly reveals our source of genuine peace and happiness in such a delightful yet helpful manner. It's a fun read—and a treasure."

—Lilias Folan, author of *Lilias! Yoga Gets Better with Age*, host of the television series *Lilias, Yoga, and You*, and known as the First Lady of Yoga

"In these turbulent times of extreme agitation, fear and overwhelm, an ocean of peace lies hidden beneath the stormy waves. Julie Lusk, Yoga Nidra mentor and master teacher, skillfully directs our attention within, guiding us to rest lightly in the natural, peaceful presence of our own deepest wisdom. To help bring healing peace to our world—inner and outer—this manual gives key instructions essential to finding "the peace that passeth all understanding."

—Christopher Baxter, ERYT 500, founding member Kripalu Center and Yoga Alliance, author of *Kripalu Hatha Yoga*

"This book is a treasure trove of Yoga Nidra scripts from the author and other noted masters in the field...You will find scripts for children, teens, men, women, or anyone in chairs, as well as a multitude of purposes and intentions. No teacher or practitioner of yoga is complete without a Yoga Nidra practice, perhaps the simplest yet most profound experience that yoga has to offer."

—Anodea Judith, PhD, author of *Wheels of Life*
and *Anodea Judith's Chakra Yoga*

YOGA NIDRA
meditations

About the Author

Julie Lusk, MEd, E-RYT-500, NCC, (Milford, OH) has specialized in yoga, relaxation training, guided imagery, and meditation for decades. An international writer, recording artist, speaker, and workshop leader, Julie is talented in bringing the best out in others through her depth of knowledge, natural light-heartedness, and caring nature. Julie's books include *Yoga Nidra Meditations: 24 Scripts for True Relaxation*, *Yoga Nidra for Complete Relaxation & Stress Relief*, *Yoga Meditations*, two volumes of *30 Scripts for Relaxation, Imagery & Inner Healing*, and *Desktop Yoga*. Visit her at JulieLusk.com.

To Write to the Author

If you wish to contact the author or would like more information about this book, please write to the author in care of Llewellyn Worldwide Ltd. and we will forward your request. Both the author and publisher appreciate hearing from you and learning of your enjoyment of this book and how it has helped you. Llewellyn Worldwide Ltd. cannot guarantee that every letter written to the author can be answered, but all will be forwarded. Please write to:

Julie Lusk
℅ Llewellyn Worldwide
2143 Wooddale Drive
Woodbury, MN 55125-2989

Please enclose a self-addressed stamped envelope for reply,
or $1.00 to cover costs. If outside the U.S.A., enclose
an international postal reply coupon.

Many of Llewellyn's authors have websites with additional information and resources. For more information, please visit our website at http://www.llewellyn.com

YOGA NIDRA
meditations

24 Scripts for True Relaxation

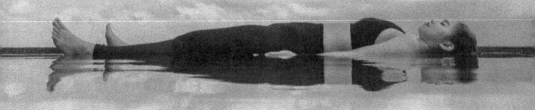

Llewellyn Publications
Woodbury, Minnesota

JULIE LUSK

FIRST EDITION
Third Printing, 2023

Book design by Samantha Peterson
Cover design by Shannon McKuhen
Interior art:
   Brain image on page 232 by Maynard Chapman, provided by the author
   Brain waves on pages 239–245 by Llewellyn Art Department
   Chakra figures on pages 16 & 234 by Mary Ann Zapalac
   Photos on pages 40–41 by Ricardo L. Ramirez
   Additional credits appear on page 281

Llewellyn Publications is a registered trademark of Llewellyn Worldwide Ltd.

Library of Congress Cataloging-in-Publication Data
Names: Lusk, Julie T., author.
Title: Yoga nidra meditations : 24 scripts for true relaxation / Julie
   Lusk.
Description: First edition. | Woodbury, Minnesota : Llewellyn Publications,
   2021. | Includes bibliographical references. | Summary: "Yoga nidra is
   an empowering meditation done lying down rather than sitting, and it
   provides the calm and focus to work through a variety of physical,
   mental, and emotional issues. This guide presents twenty-four scripts
   from master practitioners, including Kamini Desai,
   PhD, Swami Shankardev Saraswati, MD, and others. These scripts are
   developed from ancient and modern traditions, combining the best of both
   so it's easier to clear the mind, settle the emotions, and reach a
   unique state of awareness. Yoga Nidra Meditations helps foster spiritual
   development, improve stress management, and enhance physical, emotional,
   and mental health"—Provided by publisher.
Identifiers: LCCN 2020058439 (print) | LCCN 2020058440 (ebook) | ISBN
   9780738764795 | ISBN 0738764795 | ISBN 9780738765136 (ebook)
Subjects: LCSH: Hatha yoga. | Meditations. | Relaxation—Technique. |
   Stress management.
Classification: LCC RA781.7 .L8725 2021 (print) | LCC RA781.7 (ebook) |
   DDC 613.7/046—dc23
LC record available at https://lccn.loc.gov/2020058439
LC ebook record available at https://lccn.loc.gov/2020058440

Llewellyn Publications
A Division of Llewellyn Worldwide Ltd.
2143 Wooddale Drive
Woodbury, MN 55125-2989
www.llewellyn.com

Printed in the United States of America

Other Books by Julie Lusk

30 Scripts for Relaxation, Imagery & Inner Healing Vol. 1 & 2 (ed.)

Desktop Yoga

Yoga Meditations: Timeless Mind-Body Practices for Awakening

Yoga Nidra for Complete Relaxation & Stress Relief

Audio Recordings by Julie Lusk

Blue Moon Rising

Guided Mindfulness Meditations: Practicing Presence & Finding Peace

Power of Presence

Refreshing Journeys: Mini-Meditations

Sleep Well: Yoga Nidra

Yoga Nidra Essentials

Yoga Nidra: Guided Meditations for Relaxation & Renewal

Dedicated to You

Contents

Disclaimer

NEITHER THE PRACTICE OF Yoga Nidra nor this book are replacements for appropriate medical care. It is not intended to diagnose, treat, or prevent any condition. It can be used to reduce symptoms, side effects, and help with your ability to cope with your issues. If you have a serious medical condition or mental illness, consult licensed healthcare providers to get their advice before proceeding and supervise your health status as your practice progresses. The publisher, author, and contributors assume no liability for any harm caused to anyone that may result from the contents herein.

The material presented is constantly evolving. This work represents the author's current understanding and interpretation of Yoga Nidra and what the contributors have offered. The information may not represent the views of all the contributors as Yoga can be interpreted in different ways depending on the translations and source material.

The word "Yoga" can either be capitalized or in lowercase. In reality, Yoga's purpose, philosophy, principles, teachings, and all its traditions and branches go far beyond the common misperception that yoga is simply practicing postures. As valuable as postures are, it is only a fraction of what Yoga entails. Postures can be thought of as lowercase yoga, whereas capitalizing Yoga suggests a more comprehensive and accurate viewpoint. We chose to capitalize Yoga throughout this book.

Recording the Scripts

YOU MAY RECORD THE scripts for your own personal use. You may not copy or distribute the scripts to others, with or without payment, electronically, digitally, or in written form on paper or otherwise. Contact the publisher for special permissions.

Remember This

Vast and changeless,
the ground of being
is not rocked by
ripples on the pond.

The firmament from
which we spring, the
divinity at the heart
of things doesn't wax
or wane with mind states,
or wither in the wind.

We come from stronger
stuff than feelings.
Essence does not fail
or fade, diminish or
trade reality for illusion.

We are wordless, wide,
and wise beyond time.
Within us is a flame
of truth that never dies.
Let that be the focal
point of life. Let that
be the light that guides
us from the shadows.

–Danna Faulds[1]

1. Danna Faulds, *Go In and In: Poems from the Heart of Yoga* (Greenville, VA: Peaceable Kingdom Books, 2002), 81.

Acknowledgments

"Thank you, thank you, thank you," genuinely sprang from my heart each morning while writing this book. Next, the ideas and plans for the day would fall right into place and my energy would come alive. This entire project felt like an avalanche of blessings from earthly and celestial helpers, both known and unknown.

The book concept came to me while practicing Yoga Nidra early one morning. Jeanne Fredericks, my literary agent, loved the idea, guiding the process of finding the amazing crew at Llewellyn, including Angela Wix, Terry Lohmann, Hanna Grimson, and many others. Meanwhile, Jeanne and her husband were going on a cruise to celebrate a big anniversary. Not missing a beat, she took care of emails during the spotty times Wi-Fi was available on their trip. The first answers from potential publishers came in on meditation night with Amy Orr and Linda Bourquin who give me incredible love and support. Thank you, thank you, thank you.

The contributing authors are a major strength of this book. I had an ambitious wish list but no promises that anyone would help. After finally getting my nerve up to ask, I realized my apprehension was unfounded. The best people on the planet instantly and eagerly agreed to share their brilliant expertise and passion for Yoga Nidra and followed through in perfect harmony. I will always cherish the joy of getting those first yeses. Amy Weintraub was first, sending hers the day before getting married. I've been practicing Yoga Nidra with Sri

Swami Satchidananda with audios ever since the 1980s. First on cassette, then CD, and now streaming. Unbelievably, his recording had never been transcribed until it was for this book, thanks to Prem Anjali, Siva Buechner, and others at Yogaville. All the other contributors made time no matter how busy or where in the world they were, namely Rose Kress, Kamini Desai, Swami Shankardev, Robin Carnes, Stephanie Lopez, Karen Brody, Uma Dinsmore-Tuli, Jennifer Reis, and Marc Halpern. Viviana Collazo, along with her meditation, arranged for the photos of Ruth Poonawala and David Benison in savasana by Ricardo L. Ramirez. What a joyful collaboration. Everyone's support was overwhelming. Thank you, thank you, thank you.

My husband Dave is beyond amazing. He would stop whatever he was doing to help, allowing me to read him scripts. Believe me, this is not his thing. He would admit "it worked" and offer good insights. He and our dogs, Lucy and Breezy, knew right when to give me space and when I needed a hug or a playtime break. Thank you, thank you, thank you.

A tsunami of inspiration and support poured in from Cindy Lewis, Beth Owens, Mimi Sammis, Barbara Turner-Delisle, Anna and Ray Vasudevan, Albert Bollinger, Elizabeth Tenoever, Stuart McClay Smith, Caroline West, Susan Vilardo, Lilias Folan, the Nichols family, John Sawyer, Michael Arc, Christopher Baxter, Jilly Shipway, Hope Mell, John Zack, Anodea Judith, Jack Kosmach, Jess O'Brien, Danna Faulds, Nischala Joy Devi, Edwin Bryant, Maynard Chapman, and the dear women at our mornings at May Cafe. Thank you, thank you, thank you.

The members of my six weekly classes kept me on track with their encouragement and generous feedback. We were continually gratified with how helpful Yoga Nidra always was, whether it was offered live, online, or as a recording. Training people in guiding Yoga Nidra for their students, clients, and friends was profound. How inspiring to know they are offering it at hospitals, mental health centers, fire stations, big and small corporations, nonprofit organizations, where they worship, and in their neighborhoods. Thank you, thank you, thank you.

My Yoga, meditation, guided imagery, counseling, mindbody medicine, and life teachers over the past four decades are too many to name. I bow to you. Thank you, thank you, thank you.

Thank you, dear reader. May you enjoy and benefit from Yoga Nidra.

Introduction

YOGA NIDRA IS A deeply healing and empowering meditative state that starts with relaxation. It uncovers intuitive awareness, puts us in touch with feelings of unconditional peace and joy, and gives us the experience and understanding of our true nature. It is as uplifting as it is comforting and inspirational.

What a delight to write *Yoga Nidra Meditations: 24 Scripts for True Relaxation* for you, dear reader. I am overjoyed, if there is such a thing. This book had a magical feel to it right from the start. One morning, I woke up way too early and could tell that I wouldn't be falling back to sleep. Instead of getting up, I practiced Yoga Nidra, knowing it would give me a great start to my day.

I had no way of knowing how positively life changing it would be. The entire concept for this book came to me during my practice. The idea and how to implement it felt so very right. It was to be a companion to another of my books, *Yoga Nidra for Complete Relaxation and Stress Relief.* This new one would feature a collection of Yoga Nidra meditations from selected contributors and myself to provide a broad range of methods, applications, and purposes. The book proposal was written before noon. After looking it over the next day, I sent it to my literary agent, Jeanne Fredericks. She was enthused. Within a few short months, Llewellyn, a remarkable publisher, wanted to publish it.

Having something like this happen is exactly in keeping with Yoga Nidra. Part of its process sparks creativity and ingenuity. In addition, it can and will guide one's life mission and purpose through insights and intuition. The practice provides the needed energy as well.

Each contributor is top-notch and is either a highly respected author or a recording artist. Their skills have been honed as teachers, trainers, and practitioners. Many have conducted research to measure outcomes and results. They are the best. My gratitude is unending for their eagerness to share their expertise with us.

Sharing these Yoga Nidra meditations with my students and colleagues has been rewarding for all of us. Many said how uplifted they felt and how it was the most relaxed they have ever been. It's common to hear that mental chatter becomes still while time seems to blissfully disappear. Many truly gain a fresh perspective on their emotions and thinking patterns. The only complaint is that Yoga Nidra is rarely long enough!

"I get my best night of sleep after Yoga Nidra," is commonly shared, most notably during 2020, the first year of the pandemic when stress levels were especially sky high. "I feel so much happier, lighter, and content. It feels like my burdens lifted," is a frequent reaction. Many express how pain is relieved, whether from a headache or achy muscles and joints. One practitioner said, "Yoga Nidra has helped me in ways I couldn't have imagined! I've benefited from the calming of my emotions and internal chaos, using things as simple as a way of breathing, focusing on a resolve, saying a mantra, or scanning my body and allowing myself to sink into deeper levels of awareness. It mightily helped me with grieving the combined losses of my parents and my younger sister. In a brief moment during Yoga Nidra, I so strongly felt the nearness and certainty of presence of all three of them. It transformed my grief into a joy and lightness that I still treasure and reflect upon. Am I still saddened by their loss? Most assuredly—but I can call upon that totally unexpected encounter to lift me up!"

I will never forget and will always cherish my first Yoga Nidra experience. Hatha Yoga and I first befriended each other in 1975. Hatha is the aspect of Yoga comprised of postures (asanas) and specialized breathing (pranayama). Little did I know it would become a lifelong connection of practice, study, and teaching. Even though lying quietly on one's back in savasana was included back then, it wasn't until the early 1980s that I got my first real taste of deep relaxation at a conference. At that time, I was busy working professionally as a college counselor and assistant dean of students. I will always remember how completely centered, still, and peaceful I felt physically, mentally, and emotionally during a guided relaxation experience. It profoundly touched me in a beautiful manner with a bright and solid sense of spirit. From then on, this became a major cornerstone of my personal practice, study, and teaching. The expansion of Yoga, meditation, guided relaxation, imagery, and visualization were steadily integrated into nearly everything as the years came and went.

My study took another huge leap forward in the early 1990s when Whole Person Associates asked me to write two volumes of *30 Scripts for Relaxation, Imagery and Inner Healing* for them. Producing dozens of professional recordings followed. Years of being a leader in the international wellness movement and running hospital-based holistic centers gave me the opportunity of further developing and sharing even more.

In the late 1990s, *Yoga Nidra*, a book by Swami Satyananda Saraswati (Bihar School of Yoga 1998) fell into my hands and heart. I discovered Yoga Nidra was the term used for what I had been practicing and sharing with others all along. This book deepened and broadened my understanding while offering me additional techniques for experiencing Yoga Nidra. Ten years later, more enriching layers were added during my iRest teacher training. iRest, or Integrative Restoration, is an approach to Yoga Nidra that is represented in this book.

Much to my delight, New Harbinger Publications invited me to write *Yoga Nidra for Complete Relaxation & Stress Relief* (2015). This gave me the opportunity to delve even deeper into Yoga Nidra's principles, practices, and applications from the perspective of its historical roots to contemporary science and understanding. Everything came together the more I integrated the wisdom teachings from Yoga's sages with my professional training in Yoga, counselling, meditation, guided imagery, relaxation training, hypnosis, and other mindbody techniques. A diversity of students happily practiced a variety of techniques and scripts with me to discover what worked, delighting in the benefits Yoga Nidra bestowed. How fortunate that my materials have been translated into several languages to help spread the joy of Yoga Nidra and all it encompasses. This life of service has far surpassed my wildest dreams.

The practice of Yoga Nidra itself deepens and extends my Hatha Yoga experience. It serves as an effortless prelude into meditation and links these wonderful practices together. Practicing Yoga Nidra is peaceful, replenishing, and reveals intuitive knowing and guidance. It propels my journey with Spirit.

As you will see for yourself, Yoga Nidra is a phenomenal experience and offers so much in a variety of ways. It is my hope and prayer that this book will help an incredible number of people in countless ways, especially you.

About the Book

This book is for you whether you are an individual practitioner or an instructor. For ease of presentation and understanding, this book will speak directly to those of you who are just getting started on developing your Yoga Nidra practice or are interested in deepening your understanding and practice. This book is equally valuable for instructors and trainers. It will help you expand your repertoire and skills for leading Yoga Nidra in your classes, workshops, and with individuals. Information pertinent to your needs are found in appendix 4, Guidelines for Leading Others.

Part 1 is designed to get you off on the right foot. The first chapter gives you the background needed for understanding Yoga Nidra. Impressive benefits for a variety of physical, mental, and emotional issues are given. You'll learn how to make empowering and enduring behavioral and personality changes by using a self-selected intention called a *sankalpa*. Creativity, intuition, and spirituality often blossom.

Guidelines are given for personal practice in chapter two. Your questions will be answered on how to get ready for practice as well as how often and how long to practice. Guidance is given on handling distractions ranging from restless thoughts to physical discomfort.

Part 2 highlights the practice and experience of Yoga Nidra. Each meditation is meant to stand on its own so there is some repetition among the scripts. This serves to highlight each contributor's own way of expressing the material, giving you valuable insights into a variety of methods used to experience Yoga Nidra. This repetition of key concepts and practices will deepen your understanding and reinforce your memory while you are discovering your favorites. For instance, it is well worth it to devote yourself to the instructions given for savasana, the relaxation pose. Going through it every time really pays off, whether you are making minor or major adjustments. The chapters listed below will guide you through the Yoga Nidra meditations as follows:

"Foundations" (chapter three) features Nidra meditations from various styles and methods that underpin the practice and provide valuable experiences, understandings, and benefits.

"Special People and Groups" (chapter four) is aimed toward kids, teens, men, and women. Approaches taken for youngsters will differ from that taken with members of the armed forces and veterans. However, don't limit yourself. We found that adults enjoyed the one for kids, women liked the one aimed for men, etc.

"Health and Well-Being" (chapter five) is where you will find meditations appropriate for easing anxiety, depression, pain, insomnia, as well as for other health conditions. In addition, they are helpful in generating and maintaining good health in general.

"Fifteen Minutes for Yoga Nidra" (chapter six) is geared for when time is short. They still go through all the stages, but in an abbreviated fashion.

Appendices are provided to round out your understanding. Appendix 1 covers *pratyahara* and the rotation of consciousness, a technique used for sense withdrawal for healing and to relax deeply. Appendix 2 explains the chakra energy centers and their relationship to Yoga Nidra. Appendix 3 features the benefits Yoga Nidra has on the brain, including how your brain waves are affected by each stage of Yoga Nidra and the positive effects this has on your physical, mental, emotional, and spiritual health. Appendix 4 is valuable for those of you who want to lead Yoga Nidra in groups and for individuals.

A glossary and pronunciation guide are provided to fortify your understanding. Finally, resources and references are given for future study.

Quick Start Guide

Use this quick start guide to familiarize yourself with Yoga Nidra and how to enjoy and benefit from your practice. We will get into more details moving forward.

Yoga Nidra Overview in Principle and Practice

The principle of Yoga Nidra is at the heart and soul of Yoga—and of you. Yoga Nidra means *yogic sleep* in Sanskrit, India's classical and liturgical language. Simply put, it is deep restorative sleep with awareness added. It uses a systematic, progressive process that is based on traditional Yoga and backed by contemporary science to steady the mind, awaken the heart, and remove physical, mental, and emotional tension for healing and for high-level living. Doing so provides a portal for self-discovery and a trusty bridge to a wellspring of comfort, peace, and joy.

There are references in the ancient wisdom teachings of the Upanishads, classical Yoga, Puranas, and in the Tantric tradition to Yoga Nidra. Actual techniques for dependably experiencing Yoga Nidra started being developed in the mid-1970s. Additional methods, applications, and the resulting benefits continue to be advanced today.

This book gives you a variety to explore. You will find that each meditation relies on going through a systematic, reliable process to withdraw the senses (pratyahara) by releasing physical, mental, and emotional tension. (See appendix 1 for details.) As this happens, your attention begins to naturally withdraw from an outward focus to an inward one. A deeply felt sense of inner peace naturally arises.

Each meditation has a synopsis to tell you about it and a table that shows the process and methods used. The time frames given are approximate. In addition, each part of the process is identified in the script in bold, so you can easily spot them. Together, these summaries provide you a book within a book. In other words, you can use the meditation as is, or concentrate on one or more sections as you go. For instance, you may want to focus on relaxing physically or on a special breathing practice by itself. You now have twenty-four different ways to rid yourself of physical tension and just as many methods to use your breath advantageously. This gives you the freedom to customize your experience according to your needs and interests. Once you become proficient, you may want to modify and create your own sequences by substituting one method for another—just remember, the order does make a big difference. This progression is key to Yoga Nidra and distinguishes it from other meditations.

The principles and practices of Yoga go far beyond postures, as beneficial as they are. Yoga sages believe that our individual self (designated with a small "s") is made up of our personality and roles as well as our thoughts and feelings that constantly come and go. We live under the illusion that these aspects of ourselves are what is real. When we believe that these impermanent aspects of ourselves is all there is, we base our identity on an infirm foundation, like quicksand. This misunderstanding causes us to constantly search for happiness in things that do not last, resulting in having to live with an underlying sense of dissatisfaction and stress.

Our true Self (designated with a capital "S") is permanently and unconditionally peaceful, joyful, and wise. We are asleep, if you will, to who we really are. Ultimately, the goal of Yoga is to dispel this illusion by waking us up to this realization. Fortunately, Yoga's wisdom teachings have given us Yoga Nidra, one of its important and practical tools to support our well-being by waking up our awareness and important streams of consciousness. In other words, we awaken to who we really are by putting our illusions to sleep, decreasing stress, and giving us a stable and fulfilling foundation that is reliable in the long run. The experience of being beyond thinking thoughts, feeling emotions, and being tied down by our personality happens as the ego quiets. It is a place of awareness without words that is incredibly peaceful and refreshing. This enables us to live a life of meaning and purpose. Chapter one goes into more details and will aid your understanding of these important principles. If these teachings are something you agree with, fine. If not, you are invited to contemplate their meaning and implications. Rest assured; it is not necessary to accept these beliefs. Either way, Yoga Nidra still has a lot to give, as you will learn later in the book and through your personal experience.

The practice of Yoga Nidra starts with relaxation and results in profound meditation. Relaxation, one of the welcome side effects of Yoga Nidra, is the entryway and an early stage of the process. Relaxation is not the sole purpose of Yoga Nidra. Other benefits are that Yoga Nidra enables us to make durable and positive changes to our personality and make behavioral changes successfully, and it supports spiritual growth. This is accomplished by using a *sankalpa*, also referred to as making a resolve or intention. Information on sankalpas and how to make and use them is in chapter two.

Yoga Nidra is practiced lying down, usually on your back, or in a comfortable chair or bed. Powerful techniques, like relaxation training, breathing techniques, mindfulness, visualization, and meditation, are used to remove physical, mental, and emotional tension to replenish your energy and improve your overall health and well-being. All the benefits of these individual techniques, and more, are received as they build upon each other to culminate in the experience of Yoga Nidra. Refer to part 1 of the book to see some of the benefits that have already been documented. Practicing the guided meditations in part 2 will give you the actual experience of Yoga Nidra itself.

Yoga Nidra is not a substitute for proper physical, mental, or emotional health-care. Consult your health care provider. Prescription changes may be needed if your health improves. It is contraindicated for those with untreated dissociative mental health disorders, psychosis, or schizophrenia. Refer to page 256 in appendix 4 for suggestions on handling contraindications like hypertension, muscle or joint stiffness and pain, or mental and emotional health disorders with respect to Yoga Nidra.

How to Get the Most from Your Yoga Nidra Practice

Dive in. It's the actual experience of Yoga Nidra that counts. First, I recommend trying a few foundational practices from chapter one before getting into the specialized ones in subsequent chapters. To help you with this, use the overview at the start of each chapter and the summaries with each script to easily determine which ones you want to work with. Enjoy finding the techniques and methods you like and that work best for you. However, don't make the mistake of thinking Yoga Nidra is just the technique used. It can't be emphasized enough that Yoga Nidra refers to the experience of it.

Repetition pays off. You'll find that the more you experience the same meditation again and again, the more it serves to deepen and expand your experience. You'll see for yourself how each experience changes every time you practice it. However, attempting to repeat what happens from one practice to the next does not work. Instead, be open to whatever happens.

It is fun to discover that everyone has their own personal experience when practicing with others in a group, even though the meditation being led is the same. Share but do not compare your experience with other people—it varies from person to person. This provides you the trust that Yoga Nidra gives everyone just what they need.

Start a journal now. Use it to write about and reflect on your experiences. You can make notes in it on your preferences, noticing how these can change over time.

Practice Tips

- No Yoga experience is needed.

- Simply listen, participate, be alert, and accept what happens.

- Get comfy
  - Use a room where you won't be disturbed, if possible.
  - Dress comfortably. Remove anything distracting like glasses, belts, and jewelry. Empty pockets and smooth out clothing and props in advance.
  - Lie on your back. Otherwise, use a position where you are most likely to remain still and least likely to move. Examples include being on your side or sitting. Use props for support. Specifics are covered in chapter two.
  - Cover up to stay cozy and warm.

- Practice is vital. Several times a week to daily is strongly recommended, especially if you want to reap the benefits. Here is how:
  - Familiarize yourself with the instructions and meditation script beforehand and proceed on your own from memory. Specifics on things like pacing yourself with pauses are explained in chapter two.
  - Make an audio recording for personal use. Ask a friend or record yourself.
  - Get with a friend or form a group to give and receive these Yoga Nidra meditations.
  - Practice with a trained teacher. Practicing in a group often enhances the overall experience.
  - Use a professionally recorded audio. Many of the contributors have audios that are listed with their meditations. More are on the recommended resource list at the end of the book. Be careful when doing online searches for recordings. There are well-intentioned people without appropriate training who may be doing more harm than good. Check their qualifications and credentials before wasting your time.

- It's normal to tune in and out. This comes with the territory due to the levels of relaxation and awareness reached, the types of brain waves that happen during Yoga Nidra, and the internal editing that naturally and intuitively happen on your behalf.
- Plan for distractions.
  - Catch and release. In other words, catch yourself as soon as you notice that your attention has strayed, then release it, letting the distraction go.
  - Notice and investigate. Another useful option is to mindfully explore distractions by impartially observing them.
  - Relaxation-induced anxiety. If disturbed or overwhelmed, try shifting your attention elsewhere by imagining being in a safe place, or focus on lengthening your exhalation or open your eyes.
- Take your time. It takes practice to lie still, remain mindfully alert, and cultivate witness awareness. Early attempts can result in falling asleep.
- Always remember that Yoga Nidra refers to a state of awareness and not to a specific technique.

Welcome to Yoga Nidra Meditation

With all my heart, I wish you all the best in your exploration and discovery of Yoga Nidra and all it entails. You are bound to be transformed in amazing ways by these meditations. As the first lady of Yoga and author of *Lilias! Yoga Gets Better with Age*, Lilias Folan, always says, "The joy is in the journey."[2] May you enjoy every step of the way.

2. Lilias Folan, *Lilias! Yoga Gets Better with Age* (Emmaus, PA: Rodale Press: 2005), xiii.

PART ONE

PREPARATION

ONE

Yoga Nidra Essentials

A MONASTERY IN THAILAND was being relocated in the mid-1950s. While moving an ancient, almost ten-foot tall (three-meter) clay statue of Buddha, the monks saw it cracking. Just imagine their reaction. Upon peering closer, they began to see a glimmer of light emanating from the fracture. They began hammering away. They found gold inside all that clay—five-and-a-half tons of pure, solid gold. Now imagine their reaction.

Historians believe the original monastery was about to be attacked around the fourteenth century by Burmese invaders, known for stealing gold and melting it down. The monks covered the golden Buddha in clay to conceal and protect it. Thinking the statue was worthless, the intruders left it alone. Unfortunately, none of the monks survived the onslaught so no one knew the statue was golden for centuries. The golden Buddha is now in Wat Traimit, a Bangkok temple.

Just like the golden Buddha, we have a golden center too. Ours is unconditionally joyful, peaceful, compassionate, and all wise. It is eternally present and indestructible. Yogis believe it to be our true nature. Ours is concealed and has become forgotten too.

The purpose of Yoga, and other spiritual, religious, and secular wisdom traditions, is to help us remember our inherent, luminous nature and bring out the gold from within us—the gold that is in everyone, including not only you and your family and friends, but all the people you have ever met and those you have not met.

Yoga masters call this core *purusha, Atman,* or *Atma.*[3] We will use Atman, translated as the "transcendental Self" by Georg Feuerstein, PhD, the author of *The Shambhala Encyclopedia of Yoga* who says, "The Self (atman, purusha) is one's authentic identity apart from all one's roles and is deemed immortal and immutable."[4] This concept is labeled differently by its usage and according to various eras and Yogic traditions. This idea is also found in other wisdom traditions. The Judeo-Christian Bible labels it the "heart" over one-thousand times.[5] Christians refer to it as the "eternal soul." Jewish mystics name it the radiant indwelling Shekhinah. Hindus and Buddhists use "pure awareness" and it is the "Beloved" by the Sufis. Taoism calls it "Tao" and is known as "no-mind" in the Zen tradition. Others name it "emptiness," "true nature," "the infinite I am," "transcendental Self," or "the Self."

Yoga Nidra enables us to experience this overlooked side of ourselves firsthand. This is done by synthesizing the wisdom handed down from Yoga's ancient sages and sacred writings with contemporary, evidence-based mind-body techniques, methods, and practices from the fields of psychology, neuropsychology, and brain science. Yoga Nidra is a powerful and exceptional state of meditation. It uses a systematic, progressive process that starts with relaxation done lying down. An inner reservoir of mental clarity, heartfelt peace, intuitive understanding, and unconditional joy are uncovered as physical tension, restless thinking, and emotional distress fade away. Sensory experience and the thinking mind withdraw (pratyahara) to reveal one's true Self (Atman). Awareness expands beyond its normal boundaries. This is experienced as awareness without words, thoughts, images, feelings, and other sensations. It gives us the

---

3. "The word in stem form is aatman (long initial a). Since it is a masculine noun, when declined in the nominative singular it becomes aatmaa. So some people represent the word in its undeclined stem form, some in the nominative singular." Edwin Bryant, an American Indologist, professor of religions of India at Rutgers University, personal communication, October 24, 2020.

4. Georg Feuerstein, *The Shambhala Encyclopedia of Yoga* (Boston, MA: Shambhala: 1997), 265.

5. Bruce K. Waltke, "Heart," Bible Study Tools, Salem Media Group, accessed October 21, 2020, https://www.biblestudytools.com/dictionary/heart/.

profound perspective of knowing all is well within us and others, even in the midst of living through the ups and downs of day-to-day life. A blissful experience of timeless spaciousness occurs. It is astonishing.

The Spirit of Yoga Nidra

Yoga theory teaches that we are multidimensional beings composed of many layers that include our body, mind, and more. The heart of Yoga is to help us understand and embody our true Self while being in relationship with all the other dimensions and layers of our self that makes us human. These layers, or sheaths, are referred to as *koshas* and are often figuratively referred to as bodies:

Anna-Maya Kosha refers to the physical body of flesh, bones, blood, etc.

Prana-Maya Kosha refers to the energetic body of the breath, life force (prana), and chakra energy. It sustains the body and mind.

Mano-Maya Kosha refers to the mental body, or the mind, composed of thoughts, perception, concepts, ideas, feelings, emotions, and beliefs.

Vijnana-Maya Kosha refers to the wisdom body, higher intellect, the intuitive sense and direct awareness of your whole being, the space from which creativity arises.

Ananda-Maya Kosha refers to the bliss body of joy and a profound sense of contentment and fulfillment, experiencing full and complete awareness of the present moment, and experiencing witness consciousness and the art of stepping back with a deeper perspective.

Atman refers to the sense of oneself resting beyond the bodymind's contents (layers) accompanied by the spontaneous inner knowing and realization of the universal Presence and true Self. Atman is not a kosha.

We tend to believe that these layers, while important, are the components that make us up. However, due to their temporary and impermanent nature, they are thought to be an illusion and are understood to be our false self, even the blissful ananda-maya kosha. *Maya* is the Sanskrit term used for illusion.

It is believed that our true Self is permanent, eternally peaceful, unconditionally joyful, and loving at our pure indestructible core. Our true Self (Atman) is golden. Our essence is all-knowing, steady, timeless, and wise. Typically, we are unaware of this because it is covered over by the koshas. This mistaken belief about our identity causes unending cycles of discontent and stress. It leads to a self-defeating search for happiness in people, things, and circumstances that constantly come and go. A perpetual cycle is initiated of wanting, seeking, and getting (or not), a temporary pleasure that boomerangs back into searching for more.

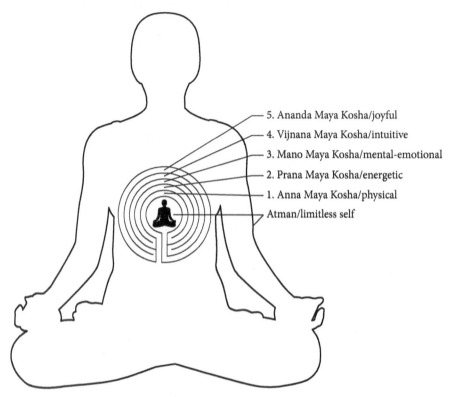

5. Ananda Maya Kosha/joyful
4. Vijnana Maya Kosha/intuitive
3. Mano Maya Kosha/mental-emotional
2. Prana Maya Kosha/energetic
1. Anna Maya Kosha/physical
Atman/limitless self

Figure 1: Atman Kosha Labyrinth

On a practical level, Yoga Nidra helps us heal, tune up, and balance each part of us (kosha) sequentially and develop skills to holistically transform stressful thoughts, feelings, and behaviors in positive ways and improve overall health. Misperceptions and limiting beliefs are peeled away, thereby shedding the illusions (maya) that cover one's true Self. This helps us get in touch with an awareness that is constant and neutral so we can enjoy the show of coming and going while living life fully, but from a point of reference that is unchanging and does not shake us up. See a wealth of benefits given later in this chapter.

The koshas can be depicted as a labyrinth with these layers surrounding, and being surrounded by, our true Self (Atman). A labyrinth is a single, continuous, one-way path to and from the center, as shown in the diagram. Walking a labyrinth and the Yoga Nidra process share similarities. First, an intention is set. Next, a clearing process takes place during the inward journey to the center. Insights, healings, peace, and Self-understanding are available while in the heart of Yoga Nidra or in the center of the labyrinth. The time of returning, the outward journey, is dedicated to integrating what has taken place along the way and for bringing the inner strength and insights gained back to daily living.

How Yoga Nidra Happens

Pratyahara, the process of training and withdrawing the senses by delving into the koshas, is at the core of Yoga Nidra practice. This is not to be confused with withdrawing from life. In fact, focus sharpens while becoming more responsive and less reactionary. Awareness expands.

Pratyahara is from the eightfold path of Ashtanga Yoga and is described in *The Yoga Sutras of Patanjali*, an ancient Yogic text. These eight components move from an external orientation to an internal one.

Ashtanga Yoga

1. Yama—(social ethics) the tenets of living respectfully with others, society, and the world include reverence for all life (ahimsa), truthfulness (satya), integrity (asteya), moderation (brahmacharya), and nonattachment, lack of self-indulgence (aparigraha)

2. Niyama—(personal ethics) the tenets for personal living and attitudes toward oneself include: cleanliness and purity (shaucha), contentment (santosha), self-discipline (tapas), Self-understanding (svadhyaya), and devotion to the Divine One, "Your will, not mine." (Ishvara-Pranidhana)

3. Asana—physical postures, poses

4. Pranayama—breath control; techniques that enhance and direct the vital life force

5. Pratyahara—training and control of the senses, sensory withdrawal

6. Dharana—mental steadiness; concentration

7. Dhyana—meditation, contemplation

8. Samadhi—absorption, super-conscious state, union with Divine Consciousness; ecstasy

Yoga Nidra and Pratyahara

According to classical Yoga, these eight limbs are the framework for realizing the true Self. Pratyahara is the most important anga (limb) in Yoga sadhana (practice), according to Swami Sivananda, a highly respected modern-day Yoga Master.[6] Pratyahara is the turning point and serves as a foundation for the higher practices of Yoga. It frees the mind by guiding and training sensory awareness. Without pratyahara and the ability to withdraw from outward focus to inward focus toward the Atman/Self, there is no bridge into the subtler meditative aspects of Yoga.

Unfortunately, the practice and experience of pratyahara is often disregarded today. People are mostly interested in either practicing postures or meditation and often think of them as independent of each other. Ignoring pratyahara is shortsighted because it diminishes the benefits of the postures and makes meditation much harder. Pratyahara naturally develops our voluntary ability to control consciousness and gives us mastery over external influences, making meditation effortless by automatically cultivating concentration (dharana), contemplation (dhyana), and union with Divine Consciousness (samadhi). This is like a beautiful rainbow that gradually changes from one color to the next.

The process of moving through the koshas to experience Yoga Nidra meditation is a pratyahara practice. It is sequential, like a time-tested recipe. The same basic ingredients (koshas) are used principally in the same order. It progressively moves from the most tangible layer (anna-maya kosha) to the most subtle layer (ananda-maya kosha) as shown in the chart below. This naturally and easily turns attention inward toward our true Self and bestows amazing benefits all along the way to the bodymind.

---

6. Sivananda, Swami, Sivananda Online, "Pratyahara," accessed June 29, 2020, http://www.sivanandaonline.org/public_html/?cmd=displaysection&section_id=893.

Like a recipe, the methods used to work with and support each kosha, as shown in the chart, can be adjusted as desired and are demonstrated in the twenty-four meditations that follow. For example, the method used for the first kosha (physical) might be progressive muscle relaxation, autogenic training, or the rotation of consciousness. Furthermore, the map used for the rotation of consciousness can also vary, as explained in appendix 1.

In addition to working sequentially with each kosha for Yoga Nidra and the experience of Atman, feel free to explore and work with the koshas individually. Perhaps aspects of yourself have been too prominent while others have been ignored or denied. Think of someone who lives in their head and ignores their emotions, or another who concentrates on their physicality while other aspects of themselves become weakened. Perhaps it would benefit you to focus exclusively on tension reduction for a while or learn ways to calm down by dedicating time to the breathing techniques.

This handy reference chart will help you pull all this together by linking these principles with the practices, their purpose and benefits, and how it likely feels as each kosha is experienced. The techniques listed are used in the Yoga Nidra meditations. The abbreviated table at the start of each meditation indicates what techniques are used for each kosha.

Yoga Nidra Practice Chart

Sanskrit Name	Relates to	Techniques to Access and Assist	Purpose and Benefits	Felt Experience
Anna-maya kosha	Physical body: Muscles, bones, skin, fluids, flesh, vital organs, etc.	• Rotation of consciousness with optional nyasa by adding a mantra/visualization at each point. See appendix 1 for clarification. • Progressive muscle relaxation techniques and variations. • Autogenic training. • Systematic stretching and tension release. • Sensory awareness. • Breathwork is sometimes used in conjunction with the above.	• Relieve physical tension to promote healing and relaxation. • Activate the parasympathetic nervous system to stimulate the relaxation response. • Deactivate the sympathetic nervous system to reduce negative effects of stress. • Bring automatic unconscious, physical functions under self-control.	• Heaviness is experienced as tension is released. • It feels like the body is sinking down and fully supported by the floor or chair.
Prana-maya kosha	Energetic body: Lifeforce that sustains the body and mind. Prana is also called chi; ki.	• Breathing techniques (pranayama). • Awareness and balancing of chakras (energy centers). • Clearing and purification of nadis (energy channels).	• Tune up the energetic body. • Bring balance between body and mind. • Thoughts start moving to the background. • Guiding voice comes and goes.	• Deep stillness accompanies heaviness. • The need to move diminishes. • A motionless feeling occurs. • Breathing deepens and slows.

Kosha	Description	Techniques	Benefits	Experiences
Mano-maya kosha	Mental body: Mind, composed of thoughts, emotions, limiting beliefs, etc.	• Experience the paradox of opposites. • Witness consciousness. • Mindfulness. • Guided imagination and visualization. • Mantra repetition. • Mentally brushing thoughts, feelings, memories away with breath. • Habituation to sensory experience. • Breathwork is sometimes used in conjunction with the above.	• Release subtle stress and tensions. • Removal of mental and emotional "scars." • Release memories and beliefs regarding injuries, etc. • Train rather than control thoughts. • Gain perspective.	• Lightness and buoyancy are experienced due to relief from not being "held down" by physical, mental, and emotional tension. • Thoughts arise and dissolve. • Imagination awakens. • Feels dreamy. • Breathing is soft and subtle.
Vijnana-maya kosha Also called Buddhi.	Intuition and wisdom. Higher intellect beyond rational thinking. Non-mental process.	• Guided imagery to welcome in and reveal intuitive wisdom. • Witness awareness. • Quiet time to allow for insights to arise.	• Relieves the intellect, ego. • Promotes detachment and distancing from thoughts and feelings. • Higher knowledge and intuitive wisdom emerge.	• Lightness. • Detachment from worldly cares. • Weightlessness. • Breathing is noticeably light.

Sanskrit Name	Relates to	Techniques to Access and Assist	Purpose and Benefits	Felt Experience
Ananda-maya kosha	Body of Joy.	• Naturally occurring peace and joy arise. • Time given for internal rest and peacefulness. • Joyful memories can be used to relive and sense joy physically. The memory is released for joyful dwelling.	• Total ease with external and internal stillness. • Very quiet. • Contentment and deep indwelling satisfaction are present.	• Bliss. • Timelessness. • Spaciousness. • Absolute stillness. • Resembles sleep but with awareness. • Physically "out of body" and into Divine blissful body.
Atman True Nature Not a kosha.	True Self.	• Time given for experiencing the essence of oneness.	• Pure Presence.	• Indescribable. • Profound contentment. • Genuine satisfaction. • Sense of oneness. • Awareness of existence beyond the body (Turiya).
	Closing.	• Bring attention back to the mindbody in reverse order. • Stretch and sit up.	• Integration. • Awareness returns to wakefulness. • Externalize. • Move the practice into everyday life.	• Feeling awake, alert, centered, grounded, peaceful and calm.

Benefits of Yoga Nidra

Benefits happen in stages. Some will happen right away while others will develop over time. Your physical, mental, and emotional well-being will improve during Yoga Nidra as your skills advance for handling stress. You will know how to recognize and release physical tension before it becomes problematic. Taking right action and developing positive qualities and attitudes is enhanced. You'll learn to welcome whatever is happening with the awareness and impartiality of mindful awareness. Your ability to calm restless thoughts and the capacity for clear thinking will grow. Decision making improves. Handling emotional distress becomes quicker and easier. What used to bother you starts fading away. Your overall sense of gratitude enhances. Appreciation for beauty and goodness come alive. All these abilities and benefits will spill over into daily life as more time is spent in each phase of Yoga Nidra.

Early on, physical tension decreases, which balances the stress response (sympathetic nervous system) and the relaxation response (parasympathetic nervous system), resulting in better health and peaceful feelings. As tight muscles relax, function, flexibility, circulation, and joint health often improve. Regulating the breath rate can be used for balancing, calming, or lifting your energy and soothing your mind.[7] Proper breathing can help improve cardiac health by improving lung capacity, heart coherence, and can help normalize blood pressure (hypertension), heart rhythm, and rate.[8] Pain relief is common as aches and pains from

---

7. Masaki Fumoto et al., "Appearance of High-Frequency Alpha Band with Disappearance of Low-Frequency Alpha Band in EEG Is Produced During Voluntary Abdominal Breathing in an Eyes-Closed Condition." *Neuroscience Research* 50, no. 3 (November 2004): 307–317, https://doi.org/ https://doi.org/10.1016/j.neures.2004.08.005.

8. Ritu Adhana et al., "The Influence of the 2:1 Yogic Breathing Technique on Essential Hypertension." *Indian Journal of Physiology and Pharmacology* 57, no. 1 (January-March 2013): 38–44, http://www.ncbi.nlm.nih.gov/pubmed/24020097; Kamakhya Kumar, "Effect of Yoga Nidra on Hypertension & Other Psychological Co-relates," *Yoga the Science Journal* 3, no. 7 (January 2005): 70–78, Yoga Publications, Hubli, Karnataka, https://www.researchgate.net /profile/Kamakhya_Kumar/publication/215451330_Effect_of_Yoga_nidra_on_hypertension _other_psychological_co-relates/links/00b49529ed404101e6000000/Effect-of-Yoga-nidra -on-hypertension-other-psychological-co-relates.pdf; Dae-Keun Kim, Jyoo-Hi Rhee, and Seung Wan Kang, "Reorganization of the Brain and Heart Rhythm During Autogenic Meditation," *Frontiers in Integrative Neuroscience* 7, no. 109 (2013): n.p., https://doi.org/10.3389 /fnint.2013.00109; Nursingh Charan Panda, *Yoga-Nidra: Yogic Trance: Theory, Practice and Applications* (New Delhi, India: D. K. Printworld (P) Ltd. 2003), 229–237.

injuries, surgeries, and impaired or aging joints are helped.[9] The immune function can increase to improve your ability to fight germs and infections as well as improve cholesterol levels.[10] Inflammation often decreases.[11] The endocrine system balances.[12] Cell repair and regeneration is enhanced. Relief can occur from symptoms and side-effects associated with cancer, asthma, reproductive health issues (PMS, menstruation, menopause, infertility, impotence), diabetes, and heart disease when used in conjunction with appropriate medical care.[13] Cortisol, a stress hormone, decreases to help with weight loss by improving metabolism.

9. Shelly Prosko, "Compassion in Pain Care," in *Yoga and Science in Pain Care: Treating the Person in Pain,* ed. Neil Pearson, Shelly Prosko, and Marlysa Sullivan (Philadelphia, PA: Jessica Kingsley Publishers, 2019), 234–256; Marlysa Sullivan, "Connection, Meaningful Relationships, and Purpose in Life: Social and Existential Concerns in Pain Care," in *Yoga and Science in Pain Care: Treating the Person in Pain,* ed. Neil Pearson, Shelly Prosko, and Marlysa Sullivan (Philadelphia, PA: Jessica Kingsley Publishers, 2019), 257–278.

10. Kamakhya Kumar, *A Handbook of Yoga-Nidra* (New Delhi, India: D. K. Printworld, 2013), 82–94.

11. Janice K. Kiecolt-Glaser et al., "Yoga's Impact on Inflammation, Mood, and Fatigue in Breast Cancer Survivors: A Randomized Controlled Trial," *Journal of Clinical Oncology* 32, no. 10 (January 2014): 1040–1049, https://doi.org/10.1200/JCO.2013.51.8860.

12. Kamini Desai, *Yoga Nidra: The Art of Transformational Sleep* (Twin Lakes, WI: Lotus Press, 2017), 240.

13. Janice K. Kiecolt-Glaser et al., "Yoga's Impact on Inflammation," 1040–1049; Candy Sodhi, Sheena Singh, and Amit Bery, "Assessment of the Quality of Life in Patients with Bronchial Asthma, Before and After Yoga: A Randomised Trial," *Iranian Journal of Allergy, Asthma, and Immunology* 13, no. 1 (February 2014): 55–60, http://www.ncbi.nlm.nih .gov/pubmed/24338229; Khushbu Rani et al., "Impact of *Yoga Nidra* on Psychological General Wellbeing in Patients with Menstrual Irregularities: A Randomized Controlled Trial," *International Journal of Yoga* 4, no. 1 (January–June 2011): 20–25, https://dx.doi .org/10.4103%2F0973-6131.78176; Rui Ferreira Afonso et al., "Yoga Decreases Insomnia in Postmenopausal Women: A Randomized Clinical Trial," *Menopause* 19, no. 2 (February 2012):186–193, http://www.ncbi.nlm.nih.gov/pubmed/22048261; S. Amita et al., "Effect of Yoga-Nidra on Blood Glucose Level in Diabetic Patients," *Indian Journal of Physiological and Pharmacology* 53, no. 1 (January–March 2009): 97–101, https://pubmed.ncbi.nlm.nih .gov/19810584/; Kamakhya Kumar, "Reversing the Ischemic Heart Disease Through Yogic Relaxation," *National Yoga Week,* organized by Morarji Desai National Institute of Yoga, New Delhi, *Nature and Wealth* 3, no. 1 (January 2009): n.p., https://www.researchgate.net /publication/215585754_Reversing_the_Ischemic_Heart_Disease_through_Yoga_Nidra.

Cortisol reduction helps memory and sleep improves. Anxiety decreases.[14] See more documented benefits in appendix 3.

Yoga Nidra and the Brain

Patanjali writes in Yoga Sutra 1.2 that "Yoga is the restriction of the fluctuations of consciousness."[15] This is exactly what Yoga Nidra does! It literally slows the fluctuation of brain wave frequencies. Beta brain waves decrease as alpha, theta, and delta brain waves increase.

During the first stage of physical relaxation (*anna*), stress is reduced causing high frequency beta brain waves to lower considerably. In the second stage (*prana*), abdominal breathing produces a rise in the "feel good" neurotransmitter serotonin as shown on EEGs.[16] Mental and emotional balance and mindfulness is the focus during the third stage (*mano*) of Yoga Nidra, which promotes alpha and theta brain waves. Mood swings and emotional distress gradually even out. Mindfulness stimulates functioning of the prefrontal cortex of the brain, promoting memory, concentration, and problem-solving while reducing anxiety and depression.[17] Creative flow amplifies when specific areas of the prefrontal cortex decrease that are responsible for sensing the egoic self, self-doubt,

---

14. Kamakhya Kumar, "A Study on the Impact on Stress and Anxiety Through Yoga Nidra," *Indian Journal of Traditional Knowledge, NISCAIR,* New Delhi 7, no. 3. (January 2008): 401–404, https://www.researchgate.net/publication/215448826_A_study_on_the_impact _on_stress_and_anxiety_through_Yoga_nidra.

15. Georg Feuerstein, *The Yoga-Sutra of Patañjali: A New Translation and Commentary* (Rochester, VT: Inner Traditions, 1989), 26.

16. Masaki Fumoto et al., "Ventral Prefrontal Cortex and Serotonergic System Activation During Pedaling Exercise Induces Negative Mood Improvement and Increased Alpha Band in EEG," *Behavioral Brain Research* 213, no. 1 (November 2010): 1–9, https://doi .org/10.1016/j.bbr.2010.04.017.

17. Neha Gothe et al., "The Acute Effects of Yoga on Executive Function," *Journal of Physical Activity and Health* 10, no. 4 (May 2013): 499–495, https://doi.org/10.1123/jpah.10.4.488; Britta K. Hölzel et al., "Mindfulness Practice Leads to Increases in Regional Brain Gray Matter Density," *Psychiatry Research: Neuroimaging* 191, no. 1 (January 2011): 36–43, https:// doi.org/10.1016/j.pscychresns.2010.08.006; Sara W. Lazar et al., "Meditation Experience Is Associated with Increased Cortical Thickness," *NeuroReport* 16, no. 17 (November 2005): 1893–1897, https://doi.org/10.1097/01.wnr.0000186598.66243.19.

and self-control. Memory improves.[18] The fourth stage (*vijnana*) is associated with theta. Creative solutions, ingenuity, and insights prosper in positive and productive ways. Yoga Nidra meditation itself happens in delta when the brain's frequency is at its slowest, yet one remains aware. Anandamide, a fatty acid neurotransmitter and endocannabinoid, naturally increases in this stage. It is nicknamed after *ananda*, the Sanskrit word for bliss, because it stimulates feeling happy. It is classed as a homeostasis regulator that helps support mental wellness.

Overall, energy replenishes, and exhaustion is eliminated. Identification with the impermanent and temporary nature of living is replaced with identifying with the golden aspect of oneself that endures—one's true Self.

Brain wave states experienced during Yoga Nidra are also the brain wave states of sleeping, the reason why it is said that an hour of effective Yoga Nidra approximates four hours of typical sleep.[19] See chapter one and appendix 3 for more on brain waves and Yoga Nidra. In addition, biological sleep only refreshes the bodymind at best and cannot enhance Self-realization like Yoga Nidra can. While Yoga Nidra is replenishing, it cannot replace sleep.

See the chart in appendix 3 for an outline of the brain waves experienced during Yoga Nidra and the documented benefits and effects this has on the body and mind.

Sankalpa: How Yoga Nidra Helps You Make Positive Changes

Yoga Nidra is fertile ground. These potent brain waves can be used to our advantage by making a *sankalpa* at the start and end of practice.

A sankalpa is a special intention, a self-selected resolve that you choose yourself. It is a sacred vow or pledge you make in support of your highest good. It is a quality that helps you become or do something worthwhile with your life.

---

18. Wolfgang Klimesch, "EEG Alpha and Theta Oscillations Reflect Cognitive and Memory Performance: A Review and Analysis," *Brain Research Reviews* 29, no. 2–3 (April 1999): 169–195, https://doi.org/10.1016/S0165-0173(98)00056-3.

19. Kamakhya Kumar, "Complete the Course of Sleep Through Yoga Nidra," *Nature & Wealth* 7 no.1 (January 2008): n.p., https://www.researchgate.net/publication/215461447_Complete _the_Course_of_Sleep_through_Yoga_Nidra; P. Pandya and Kamakhya Kumar, "Yoga Nidra and Its Impact on Human Physiology," *Yoga Vijnan, M.D.N.I.Y*, New Delhi 1, no. 1, (2007): 1–8, https://www.researchgate.net/publication/260268130_Yoga_Nidra_Its_impact _on_Human_Physiology.

Trust, calmness, or gratitude are examples. Likewise, it can reflect your true Self and be expressed as "My true nature is peaceful," or "I am a conduit of love."

We spend most of our waking hours in the beta brain wave frequency. These brain waves are not conducive to making changes due to their automatic reliance on our habits and long-term conditioning. During Yoga Nidra, we can consciously create and experience alpha, theta, and delta frequencies. When a sankalpa is embedded during delta, the unconscious mind can root out useless thoughts and behaviors and create the conditions for significant and transformative change to take root and grow. It is entirely possible to develop positive qualities, make beneficial behavioral changes, improve your lifestyle, enhance relationships, find and then follow a life direction for a meaningful and purposeful life, and support spiritual growth.

If this appeals to you, it is fine to start with a general one such as, "I am healthy in mind, body, and spirit." Some contributors suggest a sankalpa for you in their Nidra meditation to support the goals for the practice.

When developing your personal sankalpa, opt for something that has meaning and significance for you. Choosing one that you "should" make or one to please others rarely brings lasting results.

There is no hurry. Time is given during Nidra meditation for yours to reveal itself naturally instead of intellectually. This is different for everybody. In some people, one occurs instantly. For others, it takes some time. If that is true for you, trust that yours may not be ready to be revealed consciously. Have confidence that it is already unfolding on your behalf for your highest good.

Having too many sankalpas or changing it too often is counterproductive and weakens its effectiveness. Narrow it down. Being consistent will yield more than you realize, so use the same one until it becomes a living reality. For instance, if compassion is your sankalpa, it will naturally bring about patience, generosity, kindness, and other positive qualities. In another example, confidence will foster inner-strength, resiliency, faith, trust, poise, and more.

Sankalpas are typically stated briefly, sincerely, and in the present tense. Back it up with gratefulness and inner will. Word it positively and clearly. "I am courageous," or "I have abundance," or "My life is worthwhile," are examples. Use "I am patient" instead of "I am not impatient." If using "I am" seems too challenging or too mindboggling, try adding "more and more" to it. For example, "I am content, more and more."

A sankalpa is first silently said at the beginning of your Yoga Nidra experience and with your whole heart. It is repeated several times at the end. Namely, when you are totally at ease and in the fertile delta brain wave state and before coming back to full awareness. Another receptive time for your sankalpa is right on the verge of waking up or going to sleep. It also helps if you use your senses to imagine what it would be like if it were already true. Finally, set it free. Let it go by releasing any attachments to results.

Refreshing your sankalpa may be in order at some point. Let this happen from the soulful heart of intuition rather than from an ego-based, impatient, restless mind. This might occur as a wording change that feels better. Sometimes another sankalpa arises with the feeling that making a change will support your growth and development, sensing its vibration and wisdom from deep inside.

Using a sankalpa is a significant part of Yoga Nidra. It distinguishes Yoga Nidra from relaxation techniques, affirmations, hypnosis, and even most meditation practices. It is bound to make a difference. It adds depth and value to your practice as well as to your life. It truly is transformative. For example, the sankalpa of a student named Val is acceptance, one that took a while to come to him. He says it has been a lifesaver, especially when he was dealing with losing his job along with other personal and family issues. He truly believes his whole outlook has changed because of his sankalpa. As life changes, he is a calmer person and is embracing the new chapters ahead, believing and accepting that when change happens it is for good reasons. Accepting what cannot be changed is another valuable aspect of his sankalpa.

Conclusion

Yoga Nidra effectively handles everyday tension and is capable of healing deep-seated stress, which provides a wealth of health benefits. It is much more than a quick fix. It can be used for Self-realization. The best way to find out what it is all about is to experience this for yourself using this book.

TWO

Guidelines for Personal Practice

LET'S DO THIS. You really can't go wrong. All it takes is to listen, participate, stay alert, and accept whatever happens. Let go of effort, expectations, and trying to make something happen. Each time you practice is likely to be different from the last. It is also common for each member of a Yoga Nidra group to have differing reactions and experiences. That is what makes it juicy.

Please go easy on yourself. Like everything, this takes practice too. Until some skills are gained, you might experience some stress at first. It can be nerve racking to notice how busy your mind can be until you pick up on how to settle it down. Relaxation-induced anxiety can be problematic. Lying down might be uncomfortable until you know how to use props. Outside distractions can cause annoyance while learning what to do about them.

The More Consistent Your Practice, the Better the Results

Most of all, Yoga Nidra is enjoyable, healing, and downright blissful. The effects build upon themselves and are cumulative. Your skills and abilities will increase, enabling you to reach Yoga Nidra more quickly and deeply. Your resolve (sankalpa) will be reinforced as well, meaningfully coming to life and bringing with it its benefits. All these advantages—and more—will begin to spill out into your life and mindstyle. The tools you are developing will influence your energy and increase awareness. You will soon know how to calm down or lift yourself up by changing your breathing patterns. It will be easier to handle distractions and disturbances. As restlessness settles, your concentration, imagination, and creativity increase. Your emotions become more informative, manageable, and useful as your innate intuition becomes alive and well. More unconditional peace and joy will be noticed. Enhanced energy will be available to you for healing and to support having a life that is meaningful.

Periodic practice is always better than none; however, a daily practice is ideal, especially when you are under a lot of stress or are sick. A regular practice helps overcome exhaustion. This is evident when you cannot stay alert during Yoga Nidra and go to sleep. If this is true for you, resting up with Yoga Nidra and getting about eight hours of sleep nightly is important for your health. Once your energy replenishes, you will be able to stay awake and alert during the entire practice even though your body, mind, and emotions are physiologically asleep.

Choose Meditations that Appeal to You and Your Needs

A good place to start is with the foundational meditations found in chapter three. Feel free to explore all the experiences presented. Some have a more permissive flair while others are more directive in tone. Lots of variety is offered as well for each phase of Yoga Nidra. For example, you will find there are different maps used for the rotation of consciousness if that is the technique used. Some start at the mouth while others start at the hands or feet. The right side goes first in some and others start on the left. The important part is that it is effective and based on the fundamental scientific and spiritual principles underlying Yoga Nidra. Once you find the pattern you like, most recommend staying with it. The repetition will support your experience since you will be able to flow with it, cutting down on the need to concentrate. Doing so also facilitates and reinforces the healing effects of the movement of energy (prana) and enhances the brain-body connection (see chapter one and appendix 3). Occasionally, it may be useful to try another one for a change or for its particular benefits.

Don't limit yourself after you feel comfortable with the meditations in chapter three, even if they might be labeled for a special age group, condition, or purpose. These have all been used and refined by me and the guest contributors and play-tested in advance on general groups of people. Over and over, we found that people enjoyed and benefited from a wide variety of practices. For instance, older folks loved the ones geared toward teens. Everyone appreciated the ones for sleeping well and for managing anxiety or depression. On the other hand, if something does not interest you or seem to work as well, consider giving it a second or third chance before moving on.

Take your time and give each meditation a chance to give you all the benefits it offers. Discover and use the ones that have the most value for you repeatedly. Resist the urge to jump from one practice to the next. It is valuable to enjoy your favorites again and again, especially if it is appropriate for your temperament and needs.

Pacing Yourself

It is important to give yourself the time needed to experience what is happening during the Nidra meditation. Ellipses that look like three periods (...) are used throughout the meditations to indicate a brief one-to-three second pause for allowing what has been suggested to happen. Spaces between paragraphs suggest another brief pause. Spend about five to ten seconds when you see *(Pause.)* or go by the amount of time indicated. You will get the hang of this with practice.

Choose a Time of Day that Suits You and Your Goals

The best time is when you are most likely to do it. Choose a time that is compatible with your lifestyle and the rhythm of your household. Yoga Nidra will adapt itself to your needs.

Morning or afternoon practice typically gives you a shot of energy, unlike a nap that can leave you feeling sluggish. It also sets the stage for a day that is inspired by having good relaxed energy, uplifting ideas and intentions (sankalpa), and the reminder that you are much more than your beliefs, feelings, thoughts, and circumstances. It will be easier to remember to use your skills throughout the day when confronted by stress.

Practicing before bed clears out the stress from the day and is a wonderful prelude to a good night's sleep. It not only puts your body, mind, and emotions to sleep, it can help you stay asleep. You will also have tools for nodding back off if you should awaken. See the Sleep Relief meditation that is specifically designed for this.

It is best to practice on an empty stomach. Your digestion slows during relaxation and it is better not to interfere with this important biological process. This also cuts down on gas and the need to burp or fart. The more subtle aspects of the experience are easier to experience when the body is not having to digest food.

The Length of Practice Is Up to You

A Yoga Nidra practice can range from fifteen minutes to over an hour. An average practice is usually about thirty minutes. It typically takes a half hour to truly experience it, especially in the beginning. Feel free to linger along the way during meditations, taking as much time as you like. Remember, the time frames given can vary.

If time is short, you will gain from taking time to truly explore and experience parts of the process rather than rushing through to the end. In other words, dedicate yourself to physical relaxation during the time allotted. Perhaps explore the value of breathing for an entire session and save mindfulness practice for another time.

To accomplish one of the goals of Yoga Nidra of feeling replenished and rejuvenated physically, mentally, and emotionally, you may need to vary the duration of practice by either shortening or lengthening it. Investigate the fifteen-minute Nidra meditations found in chapter six.

In time, the more you practice and the more familiar you are with Yoga Nidra, the less time it will take to get into the spirit of it. At some point, you will be able to feel Yoga Nidra quickly and not need much time to go through the process. However, there are numerous benefits available to you by staying with the process, especially if you have special interests, concerns, or needs.

Find a Place with the Least Disturbances

Make it comfortable by dimming the lights, adjusting the temperature, and closing the door. Ask family members and housemates to be quiet. Better yet, invite them to join you. Put pets somewhere they will be happy and unlikely to bother you. Then again, there are stories of dogs, cats, and even birds settling down during Yoga Nidra time. One of my students was babysitting her neighbor's dog while he was away. Unfortunately, the dog missed her owner and was stressing out. This was very hard on both of them. One day, she decided to listen to a Yoga Nidra recording during the visit so she could calm herself down. She was delighted when the dog calmed down and fell asleep.

How to Stay Awake and Alert During Yoga Nidra

By now, you realize that the purpose of Yoga Nidra is to relax deeply while staying alert and aware during the entire process. Strategies for doing so include choosing a time of day when you are least likely to doze off. It helps to catch up on sleep to remedy exhaustion. Reminding yourself to stay awake at the outset is useful and can be included in your intentions.

Practically speaking, you can keep your eyes slightly open, sit instead of lying down (see "Chair Yoga Nidra" on page 85), or bend your elbow to hold your hand up. It will fall if you go to sleep and thus wake you up. Another trick is to tickle the roof of your mouth with the tip of your tongue. Go ahead and try that now.

Tuning In and Out Is Common

Do not be surprised at times when your attention drifts in and out, especially when practicing on your own or you are listening to an audio or a leader in a group. Take it as a good sign. This is normal and a characteristic of the alpha and theta brain wave states described in appendix 3. You will hear what you are meant to hear. Trust that it is natural for something to take precedence for a time while other aspects recede from awareness, retreating into the background by not being noticed or heard at all. Rest assured with confidence that you will be presented with whatever you are ready for in the appropriate time and place. When you notice that you have missed something, simply follow along with whatever is being guided.

How to Handle External and Internal Distractions

Learning to handle distractions, discomfort, and the wanderings of the mind during Yoga Nidra is good practice for being able to handle distractions in daily life. It bolsters concentration and can lower anxiety.

Distractions are not always bad. In fact, some methods welcome distractions. Let distractions be a call to return to the present moment. On the other hand, contributor Karen Brody, the founder of Daring to Rest, says she sometimes guides people to let their mind wander when they catch that happening, like she does in her Yoga Nidra meditation in this book.

Prevent Distractions Right from the Start

Familiarize yourself with the exercise so you know what to expect beforehand. Wear comfortable clothes and use the restroom in advance. Avoid shoes. Socks are fine for warmth. Close the door, turn electronic devices off, dim the lights, adjust the temperature, and prepare your props for comfort.

Acknowledge or Gently Congratulate Yourself

When you notice being distracted by things such as sounds, aches, congestion, or with fidgety thoughts, weird sensations, or emotional reactions, congratulate yourself. Instead of getting down on yourself or becoming analytical, practice mindfulness instead. Try being curious and aware. Be as neutral and impartial as possible while exploring whatever is happening. It is likely that the disturbance will fade away on its own. If it does not, take it as a signal that further exploration may be in order. Perhaps, it is necessary to make an adjustment to your body by moving mindfully. On the other hand, it may be signaling you to have that reoccurring problem taken care of by making some changes or seeking professional help.

Plan Ahead

Choose a neutral phrase to say silently to yourself each time a distraction pops up, and get in the habit of using it. This will help bring your awareness back to the present moment and away from whatever has unnecessarily captured your attention. This will prove helpful both on and off the mat.

Some examples include silently saying, "Not now, maybe later," or "Oh well." Another technique is to welcome it with a simple "Hello," or identify and name it as in "Hello restlessness," or "Welcome itchiness," then sense it and let it go. Disengage from it with an, "Oh, never-mind." Perhaps add a reminder that you are not your thoughts. Another good one is to use your imagination by mentally tossing them off a cliff or bridge or letting them go by placing them in a helium balloon or on a magic carpet to be carried away.

Try the "radio listening" technique. Let distractions fade into the background like half-listening to a radio playing in another room.

If racing thoughts take over, you may focus on something else for a while. For instance, count your blessings instead of running through your to-do list. In addition, try opening your eyes or change your breath rate to one that is calming. If you want to stop, start stretching and wake up. You can always try again later. Perhaps shorter segments will work better for you next time.

If something is troubling, reoccurring, or disorienting, do not hesitate to talk it over with someone you trust who has experience in these matters. Consider consulting with a teacher, minister, or mental health professional.

Diversions Are Different than Distractions

Diversions are when your experience diverges entirely, taking you off into another direction from what is being guided or from the intended experience. It might seem like you are going off course, but it might be that your higher Self is looking out for you by steering you somewhere else. Trust the process. The alpha and theta brain wave states of consciousness during Yoga Nidra free up creativity, intuition, self-understanding, and wisdom of the highest order, making way for dreamlike images to arise spontaneously. Your mind might start generating its own variations by adding personalized significance, guidance, and meaning.

Staying Still Versus Adjusting Your Position During Yoga Nidra

Some Yoga Nidra methods highly recommend not moving at all. Others allow for it, even encourage it by giving permission to do so during the practice. There are advantages and disadvantages for both. Moving activates the sympathetic nervous system and can interrupt energy flow. Staying still quiets the firing of the neural muscle fibers and deepens relaxation. As the body calms into stillness, mental gymnastics follow suit. However, if something is not letting up and is causing excessive discomfort, it may be best to move mindfully, rather than randomly or reactively, and then settle back in. Perhaps you will want to try using or adjusting your props differently next time.

Savasana

This is also called the relaxation pose, corpse pose, and the cozy pose.

Yoga Nidra is mostly done lying down in the relaxation or corpse pose, commonly referred to as either savasana or shavasana (sometimes the last a is dropped). Both spellings are correct. We will use savasana. It is pronounced shah-VAH-sah-nah or with the first "s": as in "sedan." Savasana does not refer to the experience of Yoga Nidra itself, just to the physical position.

Savasana is the most important Yoga posture. Other postures are done to prepare for it. Savasana should never be skipped after practicing Yoga poses. It is usually done lying down on the floor. A couch or bed can be used instead; however, doing so may put you to sleep. Some Yoga Nidra traditions highly recommend the traditional posture with little to no props. Others encourage using other positions and lots of props, like lying on one's side or sitting in a chair or against the wall. Savasana is harder than it may seem. The best position is the one where you are least likely to move and that supports good, comfortable alignment.

Use These Detailed Instructions and Handy Tips

These guidelines supplement the instructions given with each Yoga Nidra meditation in this book.

- Lie down, lining up your head, chin, and navel for good brain-body communication and energetic flow. Close your eyes or keep them slightly open.

- Have your head parallel and aligned with your body. Slightly tuck your chin toward your throat to make breathing easier by freeing constrictions in the trachea. Make sure to maintain the natural arch behind your neck. Use a thin pillow under your head if your neck is stiff.

- Soften and still the tongue to slow mental chatter. Place the tip of your tongue at the edge of the palate and upper teeth to help with not falling asleep. Another option is to rest the tongue at the bottom of the mouth. This is calming and makes it easier to breathe but might induce snoring. It can also help activate the parasympathetic nervous system that governs relaxation by stimulating the vagus nerve, a major nerve that connects all the major organ systems throughout the body. Others like to have the tip of the tongue placed softly between slightly parted teeth. Experiment.

- Move your shoulders down from your ears. Lift your shoulders up slightly and lower them back down so the shoulder blades are in good contact with the floor. Place your arms out from your sides so they do not touch your body. Having your palms up is easier on your shoulders and lowers sensory input since your fingertips are not touching anything. However, you may prefer to keep your arms closer to your body or rest your hands over your heart or belly or with your palms down.

- Notice your low back, hips, and buttocks. Move around until it feels fairly even and supported down there.

- Straighten your legs out. Rest your feet out to each side so the insides of your legs are not touching. To relax the legs, hips, and back, you may like having your feet on the floor with your knees up instead. Try using props described in the next section. Experiment.

- Finally, scan your body and make your own personal adjustments until you are so comfortable that there is no need to move at all.

- Before sitting up afterward, roll from your back to your side and rest. Use your arms to push yourself up to sitting. Doing so protects your back from unnecessary strain.

- Spend time sitting after each experience so the energy can spread, rise, and circulate.

Use Props for Comfort

Using props makes it easier to stay still and remain alert by reducing discomfort and distractions. Official yoga props are nice but not needed. Household items work well. Use the options below that work for you. Forget the rest.

- Something to lie on. A yoga mat or beach towel is fine but may not be thick enough, especially when on the floor for a half hour. For extra padding and warmth, use a thick, non-slip blanket or camping mat with your yoga mat. Being on a bed, sofa, or chair are more options.

- Support your head and neck for comfort. Use either a thin, one- to three-inch cushion or pillow under your head. A small, rolled-up towel or pillow can go behind your neck. Either way, maintain the natural arch in the back of the neck. This head and neck position helps the nervous system relax and can prevent snoring. A thick pillow puts the head and neck in an awkward position, creating upper body tension, and can hamper breath flow and circulation. Having the head too high can signal mental alertness rather than restfulness.

- Cover your eyes. Relaxation enhances significantly by the added darkness and reduction of unnecessary eye movements from the weight. Try an eye pillow, wash cloth, tissue, or scarf. Do not cover your nose.

- Support and relax your back, hips, and legs by placing a firm pillow, blanket, or bolster under your knees or under the full length of the hamstrings (thighs). Experiment with placement and different heights to find what feels best for you.

- Place something on your belly that weighs up to ten pounds such as a heavy book, pillow, or sandbag. This stimulates the relaxation response by activating the parasympathetic nervous system.

- Cover up with a cozy blanket to stay warm. At least have one handy in case you get cold. Body temperature typically drops during deep relaxation.

Alternate Positions

Use these other positions to accommodate your needs, add variety, and expand your ability to relax while in different positions.

- *Elevate and prop up your back and head.* Put a large yoga bolster, big sturdy pillow, or folded nonslip blanket beneath you. This can ease back issues and help prevent snoring. People with sleep apnea, cardiac disease, and acid reflux can benefit from elevating their back and head.

- *Rest your calves on a chair seat with your back on the floor.*

- *Lie on your side.* Support your head with a pillow and place another one between your knees to keep your head, neck, and spine aligned. Being sideways may improve airflow of the breath and may make it easier for the brain to clear out beta-amyloid, a waste product. Choose whichever side is most comfortable for you. Take into consideration that being on your left side can prevent heartburn, aid digestion, and may improve immunity. Lying on your right side can encourage calmness since it activates the right hemisphere of the brain (ida nadi).

- *Sit in a chair.* With legs uncrossed, either have your feet flat on the floor, use the footrest on a recliner, or rest your legs on another chair facing you. Place the chair back against a wall to rest your head against. Other options are to sit on the floor while leaning your back against a wall with a bolster at a comfortable angle (try 45 degrees). A neck pillow that travelers use will help support your head. Investigate "Chair Yoga Nidra" on page 85.

- *Stand* while leaning against a wall for support.

For Pregnancy

Yoga Nidra is extremely valuable during pregnancy, according to Viviana Collazo, a Prenatal Yoga specialist and contributing author.[20] Here are her recommendations to make it safe and enjoyable.

Use three pillows or cushions. Lie down onto your left side on a thick cushioned mat or bed. This posture is beneficial for all trimesters as it promotes sufficient flow of circulation to your heart, in connection to the fetus. Use one pillow for the left side of your head, another one in between your legs, and hug the third one between your arms. This brings overall postural support to your head, back, hips, and shoulders. Do not lie on your stomach.

During your first trimester, you may feel perfectly comfortable lying on your back. Follow the tips above for savasana.

---

20. Viviana Collazo, "Journey Through a Conscious Spiritual Pregnancy and Birthing" (PhD diss., Orlando, FL. Alliance of Divine Love Doctorate Program, 2009), n.p.

Try Out Some of These Savasana Options

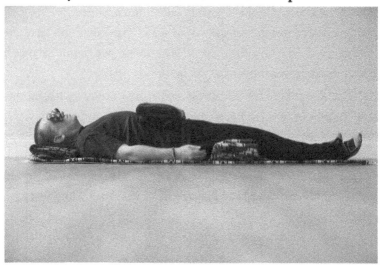

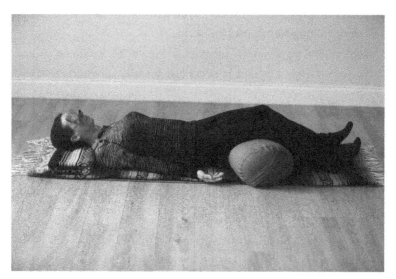

Figure 2: Savasana options

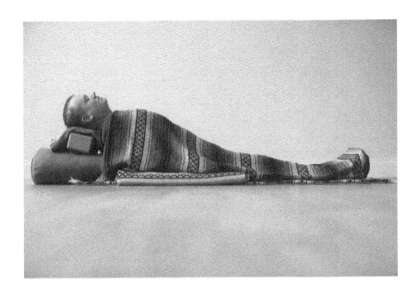

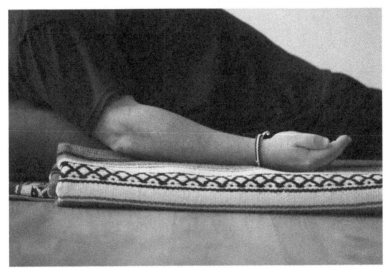

Figure 2: Savasana options continued

Let your Yoga Nidra adventure begin. While learning about it and getting prepared is important, there is nothing like experiencing it for yourself. Remember, all that is needed is to participate, be alert, and accept what happens. Enjoy!

PART TWO
PRACTICE

THREE

Foundations

THESE MEDITATIONS EMBODY THE true spirit of Yoga Nidra. They exemplify the universal principles of the practice using various methods and styles to give you valuable experiences, understandings, and benefits.

Guided Relaxation with Sri Swami Satchidananda

This progressive deep relaxation experience offers step-by-step instructions for relaxing the body and mind, calming and observing the breath and, finally, leading you to the awareness of your true nature as peace. Your body's natural healing powers are given space and allowed to rise while surrendering into deep peace.

Yoga Nidra for Genuine Freedom–Julie Lusk

Tension is washed away with waves of relaxation coursing through your body. Restless energy is calmed with segmented breathing. All this is enhanced with guided imagination using the idea of a curtain lifting on a stage for gaining perspective on the everyday world and on one's true Self. The experience of intuitive knowing and guidance awakens, paving the way for a soul-satisfying experience. A heartfelt pledge (sankalpa) is incorporated.

Total Yoga Nidra–Uma Dinsmore-Tuli

Breath awareness and placing bright little stars (nyasa) during a rotation of consciousness are the prelude for fostering creativity. Sensing the opposites of expansiveness and feeling grounded with witnessing follows. Tuning in to your heart's wisdom is included.

Heartfelt Yoga Nidra Meditation–Julie Lusk

Mindbody sensing using the rotation of consciousness relaxes and balances you holistically. *Sohum*, the natural sound of the breath, is used as a mantra. Inner eye gazing (chidakasha) further calms the mind while awakening intuition as a prelude to heartfelt imagery and inner guidance. Ample time is given for dwelling in the peaceful spaciousness of Yoga Nidra. A heartfelt pledge (sankalpa) is incorporated.

Tender Time Yoga Nidra–Julie Lusk

Progressive muscle relaxation with a light amount of tension is used instead of tensing muscle groups to their maximum. The booster breath is done by adding a pause and an extra boost after inhaling and exhaling. Mindfulness and guided imagination practice lead to feeling peaceful, spacious, and timeless. Intuition and unconditional joy often result. A heartfelt pledge (sankalpa) is incorporated

Chair Yoga Nidra–Julie Lusk

Intended for people sitting in chairs. This Yoga Nidra includes systematic stretching for tension release, focused breathing, and mindfulness to awaken inner knowing and unconditional peace and joy. The sankalpa mudra (hand position) is used to reinforce your intention.

Guided Relaxation with Sri Swami Satchidananda

Contributed by Integral Yoga on
behalf of Sri Swami Satchidananda

Time: 20–25 minutes

Summary: This progressive deep relaxation experience offers step-by-step instructions for relaxing the body and mind, calming and observing the breath and, finally, leading you to the awareness of your true nature as peace. Sri Swami Satchidananda first introduced the practice to the West in 1966 when he began teaching in Europe and then America.

As your mind adjusts to settling into Yoga Nidra, the body is reminded how to lean into itself while your internal organs begin to unwind. Blood pressure regulates, accumulated stress begins to dissipate, adrenal glands are soothed, and breathing slows and deepens. This soothing practice is also effective in dealing with insomnia. Your body's natural healing powers are given space and allowed to rise while surrendering into deep peace. It is suitable for anyone and any situation in which you can relax deeply.

Stages	Process / Techniques
Preparation and settling in	Savasana
Sankalpa	True and lasting peace and happiness
Physical: Anna-maya kosha	Progressive muscle relaxation with lifting and dropping portions of the body and breathwork
Energetic: Prana-maya kosha	Breath awareness
Mental: Mano-maya kosha	Mindful awareness

Stages	Process / Techniques
Intuitive: Vijnana-maya kosha	Witnessing of inner joy and awareness of one's true nature
Bliss: Ananda-maya kosha	Transcendental peace and joy
True Self: Atman	Awareness and witnessing true nature
Sankalpa	Rejuvenation, healing, and witnessing
Reawakening and closing	

Preparation and Settling In

You are about to embark on an experience of deep relaxation that I hope will help you to get in touch with your own inner peace—the "real you."

Every human being longs for true and lasting happiness; the path or means through which he or she attempts to find it varies according to the level of the individual's development. True and lasting peace and happiness can only be attained through the knowledge of the permanent, or Divine, which is the indweller of all beings and the source of all life. It has been given such names as the Self, Nature, God, Cosmic Consciousness, and so on.

The body, emotions, and intellect must be developed to a level in which they function healthily and in perfect harmony with each other. Only then can one live a happy and peaceful life and use them as tools to transcend limitations and to experience the Divine. To experience this inner peace, the body, the breath, and the mind, must all be in harmony. And, by keeping your thoughts in the here and now, your awareness will become more focused, and you will begin to feel more peaceful.

Deep relaxation is a simple yet highly effective technique for putting the body, breath, and mind into a state of deep relaxation. This is done in a natural progression through alternately tensing and relaxing all the muscle groups of the body. As the body becomes more relaxed, the breath and the mind also become more tranquil, allowing you to sink deeper and deeper into your natural state of inner peace.

To prepare for this profound relaxation experience, you will need to find a clean and quiet place where you can leave all your cares and concerns behind. Lie down on your back on a comfortable but firm mat, or on your own bed.

You are going to have a most beautiful experience, a very deep relaxation. Lying on your back, have your legs about a foot apart. Let your arms be relaxed and about a foot away from your sides, with the palms facing toward the ceiling. You may now shift your body slightly until you find the position that is absolutely comfortable and most restful for you. (Pause.)

Progressive Muscle Relaxation with Breathwork

This is a form of relaxation and meditation. Now, close your eyes and listen carefully to my instructions. These instructions are only a guide to help you relax and focus your awareness.

You will purposely be tensing and relaxing each part of the body. You will find that you receive maximum benefit from this if you put all your attention into each part of the body as you tense and relax it.

When I tell you to raise a part of your body—for example, your right arm —please raise it slightly, perhaps six inches or less. Then, when I tell you to release, just let that part fall to the floor, as if it were attached to a string held from above and the string had just been cut.

Let's begin.

First, have a few slow, deep breaths. Every time you inhale, feel that you are filling your body with total peace and tranquility. Each time you exhale, feel that you are blowing out all the tension in your body and mind. Inhale fresh, cool air. Exhale hot, tense air.

Now, bring your total awareness to the right leg. Inhale deeply. Tense every muscle in the right leg. Raise it a few inches, hold, and tense a little more ... and *release*. Good. Now, gently roll the leg from side to side ... and then leave it relaxed. Just forget the right leg completely. Good.

Now, bring your awareness to the left leg. Inhale, tensing the leg. Lift it slightly. Hold it tight there, tighter still, and ... *release*. Now, gently roll it from side to side a few times ... and leave it relaxed.

Now there is no tension anywhere from the hips down to your toes.

Become aware of the buttocks. Tense them. Inhale and hold the breath while tensing. Keep tensing. When I say to release, let the tension in your buttocks and your inhalation also be suddenly released ... *release* ... Good.

Now, think of the abdominal area. Take a deep breath in. Imagine that your stomach is like a balloon. Fill it with air and let it expand to its limit. Hold the breath, and when I tell you to release it, let the air burst out through the mouth ... Now, *release* ... Very good.

Now, come to the chest area. This time, inhale and fill up the chest. Let your chest expand as much as possible. Hold the breath ... and *release* ... Good.

Let's move on to the arms. Think of the right arm. Stretch out the right arm. Spread out the fingers of your right hand. Tense. Now make the right hand into a fist. Make it really tight. Inhale and raise the arm slightly ... and *release*. Now, gently roll the right arm from side to side and then, with the palm facing the ceiling, let it be.

Bring your awareness to the left arm. Stretch out the left arm. Spread out the fingers of your left hand. Now, make the hand into a fist. Make it really tight. Inhale and raise the arm slightly ... and *release*. Now, gently roll the left arm from side to side and then, with the palm facing the ceiling, let it be.

Become aware of your shoulders. Tighten your shoulders without moving any other part of the body. Let the shoulders be lifted and pulled toward your ears. Hold them tense and tight ... *release*. Once again, lift your shoulders and squeeze them tightly ... *release*. That's good.

Now, let's come to the neck area. Slightly roll the head to the right and then slowly to the left. Do this a few times and, as you roll the head, imagine that you are relaxing each and every muscle in your neck. Gently rolling, and now leave your neck relaxed and head centered.

Let's relax the facial muscles. First, open your mouth slightly and stretch the jaw from side to side. Open and close the lower jaw and move it around. And now, leave it relaxed.

Press the lips together tightly ... and *relax*.

Now, tense and wrinkle the nose ... and *relax*.

Now, close the eyes and tightly squeeze your eyes and forehead ... *relax*.

We will relax all these muscles once more by now tightening all the muscles in your face, squeezing them into a tight prune face. Squeeze more ... and *relax*.

That's it! We have literally relaxed all the muscles of the body.

Let's check once more for any remaining tension.

Without moving any part of the body, just mentally review each part, starting from the toes and moving upward, part by part: through the lower legs and now the upper legs.

If you become aware of any tension in any part, mentally repeat the word, "Relax," and feel the tension slip away...Good.

Now, we will continue by mentally checking the buttocks...the abdomen ...the chest...the lower back...the upper back. Now, checking the hands and the arms...the shoulders and the back of the neck...the face...and, finally, the top of the head.

The entire body is now completely relaxed. Your muscles are so relaxed that they might not even want to move. This is the state of deep relaxation. Take this moment to experience how totally relaxed and peaceful your body feels. *(Pause 1 minute.)*

Breath Awareness

Because of the total relaxation of the body, you do not need to breathe heavily. Your breathing is, in fact, very shallow. So, simply become aware of the breath. See how calm it is as it flows in and out, gently and rhythmically. Now you have forgotten the body and are thinking of the breath. *(Pause 2 minutes.)*

Mindful Awareness

Now, forget even the breath. You are entering an even deeper state of relaxation. Bring your awareness now to the mind. You will see that even the mind is very calm and quiet. Just allow the mind to rest. Let the mind sink into a still deeper state of rest and peace. If any thoughts come that try and pull you from the here and now, do not get involved with them. Watch them come and watch them go. *(Pause 1 minute.)*

Witnessing of Inner Joy and Awareness of One's True Nature

As the mind rests, the breath is calm and the body totally relaxed. You are able to transcend the body, breath, and mind now. You are in a transcendental state of profound peace and relaxation. Realize that this peace that you are now experiencing, as you sink deeper still into total tranquility, is your true nature. You are not the body, not the breath, nor the mind. You are only an observer, and you possess the body, breath, and mind. These are your vehicles and instruments, and you make use of them in your daily life of dedication in service to the Divine.

Remain in your true nature for a while. Enjoy this supreme peace. This is the real you. This is Self-realization. *(Pause 5 minutes.)*

Om ...

Now, allow your mind to think of the breath *(Pause.)*

Rejuvenation, Healing, and Witnessing

The entire body and mind have listened to you and they are totally relaxed. This is the best possible opportunity for the body and mind to be healed. They will be rested, revitalized, rejuvenated, and rebuilt now. Proper rest and relaxation are the best remedies for rejuvenation and healing.

As you observe this phenomenon of how you can be a witness to the body and mind, you are able to know who you are—that Divinity, the Self that transcends the body and mind. You can continue in the reality of the Self even after the body and mind come out of this deep state of relaxation. That means that you will retain this experience of who you are and you will be able to witness the body, mind, and emotions as your instruments.

You are the eternal witness. When the mind is unhappy, you are not affected by it. If the body is ill, you are not affected by it. In your waking state, even in the midst of all your daily activities, you are retaining this awareness that you are the witness; that way, you are able to raise above all situations, all emotions, all upsets in life. You will retain this awareness of who you are.

Reawakening and Closing

Now, you feel a sincere desire to make use of the body and mind in a new way. As you come out of this state of relaxation, you will retain this experience of inner peace. The body and mind will feel totally new, totally fresh, and filled with health and vitality.

Notice that your breathing is very, very slow. Now, begin to make the breath a little deeper. Slowly inhale and exhale, becoming more and more conscious of the breath. Make the breathing deeper still. As you inhale, feel that fresh energy, vital energy is flowing all through the veins—all through your body, from head to foot. This energy is energizing and awakening the entire body, part by part.

As the energy flows, you'll begin to feel a slight tingling sensation all over the face and then through the torso. Feel it moving through the arms. Feel the entire body begin to be awakened by this flow of fresh energy. Allow the energy to flow into your legs. You are able to feel the fresh energy flowing and surging all over the body. You can gently begin to move the body by stretching gently. Feel the freshness and vitality of the body.

You can now slowly and gently get up and face the day with a renewed sense of peace and joy, love and light.

Om shanti, shanti, shanti. Peace, peace, peace be unto all.

Sri Swami Satchidananda is one of the most beloved Yoga masters of our time. The founder of Integral Yoga International, he shared his vast practical wisdom and spiritual insight with seekers worldwide. His message of peace—within and without—and harmony among all faiths is more relevant today than ever. Visit SwamiSatchidananda .org and IntegralYoga.org for more.

Resources

Websites
swamisatchidananda.org

integralyoga.org

shakticom.org/products/yoga-nidra-guided-relaxation-affirmations-for -inner-peace

Books and Recordings
Integral Yoga Hatha by Sri Swami Satchidananda, Integral Yoga Publications, Buckingham, Virginia, 2017.

Guided Relaxation and Affirmations for Inner Peace with Sri Swami Satchidananda, Integral Yoga Media, Buckingham, Virginia, 2007.

Yoga Nidra for Genuine Freedom

Julie Lusk

Time: 45 minutes

Summary: This meditation is designed to lift your awareness from the mundane world to one that is supremely pleasant and free. Shifting one's perspective by progressively withdrawing awareness from the senses (pratyahara) is one of Yoga Nidra's secrets for doing this.

Being overloaded by everyday life and the constancy of sensory experience is exhausting. The ego could use some freedom by airing out and would benefit from some well-deserved rest. However, this is like putting a child down for a nap. Typically, they will fight it at first but will feel refreshed afterward. As the ego eventually quiets, attention automatically and naturally turns inward toward one's true Self: our innate, enduring source of inner peace and happiness.

A whole new world of experience is revealed. It is like opening the curtains on a stage at a playhouse. The familiar side of the stage is the material world. This is the body-bound, ego-driven, constantly changing experience of mental and emotional ups and downs that continually changes from one moment to the next. What has been on the other side of the stage has been there all along but has gone unnoticed due to focusing on everyday life. Lifting the curtain reveals a constant, all-pervasive sanctuary of well-being that is one's true Self. Energetic awareness is free to move inward where there is an infinite source of uplifting, restorative calmness that can be used to remove illusion and supercharge oneself.

Yoga Nidra is designed to give you access to the entire stage. By lifting this curtain, so to speak, you can go back and forth from the land of doing, thinking, and feeling to the land of wisdom, peace, and bliss. Once these dimensions of oneself are harmonized and reunited into wholeness, we can use the spotlight of friendly awareness for focusing more clearly on what's important. Eventually, we can live comfortably on the whole stage of doing and being, giving us a healthy perspective for Self-understanding and living life fully.

This process happens in stages. In this practice, the imagination is used to wash physical tension away and replenish life force energy (prana). This new-found energy is dispersed and available for healing and renewal, both through-out the meditation and afterward (prana dharana).

Next, the breath is used for energy enrichment, distribution, and balancing. Cultivating the capacity for effectively handling distractions and to pay attention are nurtured.

In the next stage, the restless mindbody settles down as the brain gets tired and bored with paying openminded attention to present-time environmental and sensory cues, such as listening to ambient sounds. This is called habituation. It frees more energy on your behalf by providing a safe container for being mindful and attentive with presence. The thinking, judging mind can go offline for a while when mindfulness is in the forefront. The tranquility of awareness without words results, enabling us to enjoy life with fewer distractions and helping us live life with more ease no matter what is happening.

All this is enhanced with guided imagination by using the notion of a curtain lifting to reveal the entire stage of a playhouse. The world of thoughts, feelings, objects, and actions are recognized as actors coming and going on the stage of awareness. Watching what is happening from the audience is akin to witness awareness. Like an intermission, learning to rest with open awareness in the often-unrecognized gap between thoughts is refreshing. This is simply relaxing with panoramic attention with no specific object of concentration or attention (breath, sound, gaze, etc.). The experience of intuitive knowing and guidance awakens, paving the way for a soul-satisfying experience.

A heartfelt pledge (sankalpa) is utilized at the start and end of the practice.

Additional Notes: This is written for someone who is lying down. However, it can be done in a prone, side, sitting, or standing position.

Stages	Process / Techniques
Preparation and settling in	Savasana
Sankalpa	Heartfelt pledge

Stages	Process / Techniques
Physical: Anna-maya kosha	Body tension is eased away with imagination, sensory awareness, and habituation
Energetic: Prana-maya kosha	Segmented breathing emphasizing a three-part exhalation
Mental: Mano-maya kosha	Guided imagination with the concept of a stage is used
Intuitive: Vijnana-maya kosha	Experiencing intuition
Bliss: Ananda-maya kosha	Joyful rest
True Self: Atman	Pure awareness
Sankalpa	Heartfelt pledge
Reawakening and closing	

Preparation and Settling In

Let's have a delightful Yoga Nidra experience. Make yourself as comfortable as possible. Being at ease physically helps to calm your mind into stillness, enabling you to discover an inner oasis of overall well-being.

Begin getting comfortable, allowing your body to rest for now... settling in more and more... It helps to have your nose and chin in alignment with the center of your chest... Next, gently move your shoulders down from your ears, tucking your shoulder blades underneath so your upper back feels nice and supported... Have your arms a comfortable distance away from your body with your palms up...

Take a big breath in and sigh it out... Adjust your mid-back and low back for more stability and comfort... For more back and leg comfort, move your feet about a foot or two away from each other... Feel free to make your own adjustments so you're as comfortable as possible... Take another big breath in and sigh it out...

If you like, imagine yourself being surrounded by a circle, a sphere of protection. This can be made of whatever you like. For instance, this protective place might have a wall, a dome, some special things, or perhaps a group of protectors. In your own way, go ahead and activate your own security system to shelter you from harm and for safekeeping, and shielding you with loving protection... This protectiveness is always available for you whenever it's needed, like during this practice or during your day.

You may notice something calling out for your attention. Without changing it, go ahead and spotlight it with friendly awareness. Give it center stage. It could be either something that feels like discomfort or comfort, just so it's something that's happening now, grabbing your attention. Perhaps it's an area where there's tightness or tension, maybe some soreness. You may choose an area of comfort, such as where you're feeling supported or an area that feels cozy and warm.

Zero in on it for now rather than trying to ignore, change, or fix it... Give it your full attention, noticing what's going on, allowing it to be left alone while also being held by friendly unbiased attention... What are you noticing right now?... Is it staying the same or shifting and changing on its own?... What's happening?... If needed, go ahead and take care of it according to its needs. (*Pause.*) Take a big breath in and sigh it out...

Please open your eyes a little and look gently and softly at something nearby. Once your vision settles on something, there's no need to glance around or even blink, just steadily and softly gazing... Blink whenever it's needed and continue gazing... Now, blink and flutter your eyelids quickly several times... and close your eyes...

Start pressing your tongue up into the roof of your mouth or against the back of your teeth... and release... You may softly place the tip of your tongue at the edge of the palate and upper teeth to help with staying awake and aware. Try it... Another option is to have the tip of the tongue placed softly between slightly parted teeth. Try it... This time, rest the tongue at the bottom of the mouth. This is calming and can make it easier to breathe. Try it... It's your turn to experiment, choosing where you like having your tongue... It's time to soften and still the tongue to slow mental chatter way down. The softer and quieter your tongue becomes, the more still your mind becomes. (*Pause.*)

Listening now to whatever you might hear in the far distance... impartially allowing the sounds to come to you... there's no need to name them whatsoever, simply listening to the distant sounds for a while, practicing awareness without words. (*Pause.*) And being mindful and impartially aware of the nearby sounds for a while. (*Pause.*) Remind yourself to continue listening while your awareness grows, allowing your sense of well-being to flourish.

Heartfelt Pledge

Let's personalize your practice and give it more meaning and focus by using a sankalpa by making a heartfelt pledge. This happens by having an intention, a dedication for your practice. It also expands the benefits of your practice into daily living. This is a quality or characteristic like confidence or calmness. It's personal to you, perhaps something that supports your life path in meaningful ways. An example is, "I am peaceful, more and more."

Feel free to ignore this if it doesn't appeal to you or the time isn't right. Trust that whatever is in your best interest is already happening.

If you're interested, you're invited to do this now. Stay with the one you've established or invite one to take shape, perhaps appearing as a word or phrase or an image, arising from your heart of hearts, from your soul. (*Pause.*) Word it briefly, positively, and in the present tense … Silently say it to yourself a couple times with sincerity and conviction. (*Pause.*)

Feel free to take a big breath in and let it all go.

Relaxing Rhythms

Begin noticing the touch of your clothing against your body, feeling its touch and texture on your skin … Feel free to make adjustments so you're more comfortable and settle back in … Take a moment or two to feel the touch of air on your skin …

Let's rinse away bodily tension with waves of relaxation. Let a rhythm that's calming for you take shape. This could be the soothing rhythm of waves washing back and forth. It might be a gentle breeze or gently rocking in a chair or hammock. It's up to you so long as it's got a nice, ongoing rhythm that's calming and soothing for you.

And the first place you notice this gentle rhythm is your breath, allowing it to be just as it is. It's your very own rhythm; it's effortlessly you, knowing there's nothing to do now but to relax into the gentle rhythm of your breathing … The energy of your breath, your life force, begins to travel, bringing its magnificence wherever it goes.

And now you notice a gentle, soothing, relaxing rhythm happening at your feet; feel this rhythm of relaxation massaging and easing tension away ... and now it's bringing relief to your ankles ... It travels to your lower legs, helping them soften and melt into what's below ... This easy-going rhythm is washing tension away with lapping waves of comfort ... This nice rhythm is surrounding your knees ... and your upper legs are so happy it's their turn to be rinsed and refreshed ... This calming, healing rhythm is tenderly surrounding your hips ... and now it's spreading and comforting your low back; tensions are being massaged away ... Your entire back is so happy that it is its turn to receive comfort and ease, and your back is feeling fully supported now and sinks in even more ... This delightful, soothing rhythm is now going deeper inside and harmonizing your internal organs in healing ways, softening completely ... It begins flowing to the top side of your body with a beautiful gentleness ...

Feeling the easy-going rhythm of your breathing as it fills you up with peace. It's getting more and more peaceful with each gentle breath ... Peacefulness is flowing all around now and rippling out ...

Your heart is so glad now that this soothing rhythm is so comforting, and the tempo of your heart is beating happily, deeply within, in perfect unison with everything else ... Your shoulders get to enjoy all this special attention, all across your shoulders ... In your own time, this easiness begins its journey to your upper arms ... It pours down into your lower arms ... Your wrists and hands are so excited to receive the massage of this wonderful energy. Your hands feel so taken care of with this soothing rhythm ... You can begin gently opening and closing them with a very easygoing manner, slowly and softly moving your hands in their own rhythm until they completely come to rest ...

This energy flows up to your neck, inside and out, enjoying being cared for by this soothing rhythm ... This wonderful relaxing rhythm feels great as it comes to your face ... Your jaw, mouth, and tongue welcome in this beautiful energy that is relaxing and feels so softening and calming, melting completely ... Feeling your breath coming and going at an easy pace that is so natural and feels so good ... Every breath pulses with peacefulness ... And your eyes are enjoying this and happily being taken care of with the ongoing rhythm that is so soothing and comforting ... Your forehead is gently and happily enjoying the comforting massage and being soothed, more and more ... and it flows throughout your whole face ...

It's starting to go wherever it's needed now, this soothing rhythm that's so relaxing and calming, giving its comforting gifts of healing and renewal, so relaxing and restoring. (*Pause.*)

If you like, feel free to move around and settle back in.

Breathing

Every breath pulses with peacefulness... Begin listening to the sound of your breathing as it effortlessly comes and goes... sensing its tempo, letting it be just like it is...

Whenever you notice your attention has scattered, simply refocus, spotlighting your attention upon your breath, following its passage in and out gently and in its very own pattern. (*Pause.*)

Let's play with the exhalation for a while. Here's how. Begin to breathe out in segments. In other words, breathe out a little and pause midstream, breathe out a little more and pause. Keep on going until your lungs have emptied and welcome in a fresh new breath.

Please begin, breathing out in segments until your lungs have emptied out. In its own time, welcome in a fresh breath. (*Pause about 15 seconds.*)

Now, let go of that and simply breathe out naturally for a while, resting in the natural and normal pause that happens after breathing out. It's fine to rest in the space at the end of the exhalation awaiting the new breath to naturally arise. (*Pause.*) Not thinking about breathing but experiencing it as sensation, the felt experience of arising and dissolving... Soft tongue. (*Pause.*)

Quieting Mentally and Emotionally

Can you notice thoughts, beliefs, and feelings and how they are coming and going in waves?... Aware of how they come for a while as if they're an actor stepping out onto a stage at a playhouse. They stay for a while, play their part, and then leave. Always changing.

Like an intermission, take a break from the action for a sweet, quiet gap between acts where there is open, spacious awareness for resting completely.

Ever present. You can rest in the spacious gap until the next act appears. Each time this happens, they're noticed with friendly, detached awareness... Feel free to name or label whatever happens. For example, they could be called "planning," "concerns," or whatever... Perhaps it's "restlessness" or maybe "contentment." Sounds could be labeled too, like "traffic," whatever it is. Rather than analyzing, label it "analyzing."

You can shift to simply watching the play of awareness as if you're in the audience as thoughts and feelings come and go from the stage. After noticing and naming, gently return to the present moment, like to your breathing, or having a soft tongue hovering quietly within, or to the spacious gap.

Notice how this stage is an always changing field of awareness, composed of the world of thinking and doing, of dramas and comedies. You can get involved and act it out, play the part for a while, enjoy the restful gap between acts, or watch the show from the audience. (*Pause.*)

Somehow, there's a curtain that starts coming alive. Becoming more aware of what this curtain is like, noticing what it's made of... what its texture is like... what color or colors it has... noticing more and more about it...

Like magic, the curtain begins to lift, dissolving into thin air, revealing a peaceful haven, an all-pervasive refuge that's been there all along. It's so stabilizing and constant. (*Pause.*) It feels expansive, like the enormity of the ocean, the vastness of the sky. Connecting with it. (*Pause.*)

You're welcome to explore; be inquisitive with friendly awareness... Freely moving back and forth between the changing land of thinking and doing to the unchanging land of being, all the while with awareness. You're free to step off the stage into the audience, watching what is happening on the stage of life and giving you the opportunity to watch and observe what you want to pay attention to... Witnessing and watching. (*Pause.*)

Intuitive Awareness

Your heart of imagination comes alive. Inner guidance, insights, creativity, clarity, and wonder are here for you. (*Long pause.*)

Joyful Awareness

There's an undeniable sense of well-being and safety that's here, sheltering and comforting you... sensing contentment and peacefulness with the nature of things. (*Pause 1–2 minutes.*)

Pure Awareness

This is the realm of an ever present, all-pervasive, pure awareness. (*Pause 1–2 minutes or longer.*)

Heartfelt Pledge

Within this potent field of awareness, begin letting your heartfelt pledge (sankalpa) float into your awareness. It rises from a genuine place that's always in support of your overall well-being. Stay with the one you've established or invite one to take shape, arising from your heart and soul... Say it silently to yourself several times with confidence and heartfelt conviction... Imagine it taking shape in your life, more and more... Start imagining how it looks and sounds and feels. (*Pause.*) Take a big breath in and let it all go.

Closing and Reawakening

It's time to gradually return to the land of doing, knowing there's always an ocean of bliss that's always present that resides within. It's your true nature, your true Self...

Now, take your attention to your breathing... noticing your breathing just as it is for a little while... Next time you inhale, let it fill you up more and more, breathing more deeply, time and time again... Feeling the air in your nostrils throughout the length and breadth of it... noticing how this effortless rhythm fills up your lungs each time you breathe in and how your lungs empty each time you breathe out... Allowing the flowing breath to awaken you, more and more... starting to feel more alert and aware, clear headed.

It's time to begin transitioning back to this time and space, to the here and now... Begin becoming more aware of your own presence that pertains to where you are...

Aware of whatever is below you, feeling the support of the surface you're on, having a direct experience of it. Noticing the contact points as your body touches whatever is beneath you... And becoming more aware of whatever is around you, the walls, the things that are by you... and what's above you, the ceiling, the sky... Remembering, sensing wherever you are right now.

Feel free to start moving your hands or feet... and let them rest... Start moving your whole entire body however you want, moving naturally and noticing your body, more and more. (*Pause.*)

If you've been sitting, continue your experience for now. If you are lying down, please roll over onto your side and curl up, if you like. (*Pause.*)

From your side, use your arms for support to lift yourself up to sitting and settle back in. (*Pause.*) Sitting helps integrate your experience and allows your newfound energy to flow, distributing itself, going up and down your body and spreading all around... Let your hands comfortably rest. (*Pause.*)

Close your eyes, savoring your experience of inner peace, freedom, and contentment... Open your eyes a little, blending and merging the inner world with the outer world... Play with this experience of having your eyes open or closed, yet aware of blending and merging your inner and outer experience... Now, keep your eyes open... feeling more awake and aware. Ready to benefit from your experience for your own sake and for the sake of others.

Peace, peace, peace. (Om shanti, shanti, shanti.)

Total Yoga Nidra

Contributed by Uma Dinsmore-Tuli

Time: 25 minutes

Summary: This practice embodies the Total Yoga Nidra method with the intention of nurturing creativity. This was spontaneously improvised and integrates many forms of Yoga Nidra. In particular, guided imagination is used during breath awareness. The practice of nyasa is offered by using the imagination to place tiny stars throughout the body during the rotation of consciousness. An expansive yet grounded experience is fostered.

Stages	Process / Techniques
Preparation and settling in	Savasana and breath awareness
Sankalpa	Welcoming creativity
Physical: Anna-maya kosha	Rotation of consciousness with awareness of placing stars throughout the body (nyasa)
Energetic: Prana-maya kosha	Breath awareness with guided imagination
Mental: Mano-maya kosha	Expanding mindful awareness
Intuitive: Vijnana-maya kosha	Sensing creative awareness
Bliss: Ananda-maya kosha	Expanding awareness progressively
True Self: Atman	Implied experience
Sankalpa	Welcoming creativity
Reawakening and closing	

Preparation and Settling In

Welcome home to yourself. Welcome to this practice of Yoga Nidra with the intention to welcome a space for creativity. Welcome!

It's time to get comfortable. Lie down on your back. Take time to arrange yourself so that you feel that you are well supported. Place cushions and pillows under your head and wherever else suits you so that you can feel absolutely at ease. Having support underneath the knees can really help to let the lower back settle well. Since body temperature may drop during the practice, cover yourself with a blanket, or put on socks or a sweater to keep warm. Make whatever adjustments are necessary so that you feel super comfortable.

Let's begin. Settle in and allow the body to become still so there is no need for any further physical movement during this practice. If the desire to move does arise during the practice, simply watch it. It will probably go away, and you can remain still. If the desire to move returns, do so with awareness and return to comfort and stillness with zero desire for movement.

Now become precisely aware of the position in which you are lying…Know the shape and the posture of the body; know the shape and arrangement of the room. Feel the points of contact between the body and whatever you're lying upon.

Breath Awareness

Be comfortable…Notice the breath going all the way down to the very end of the exhalation and all the way up to the height of the inhalation. Welcome the full cycle of every breath as it goes all the way down to the depths of the exhalation and then all the way up to the heights of the inhalation for a few breathing cycles. *(Pause.)*

Welcome each cycle of breath as if each breath were breathing you, as if the rhythm of the breath is like the cycle of a full day as it spans from morning, noon, to night. Each breath coming in is like the dawning of the day. The height of the breath is like the noontime, bright and full. And it's like the evening as the breath begins to leave. And then, the end of the exhalation, is like the nighttime of the breath, a time of rest, waiting, and quiet until a new breath dawns, ascending to the noontime, afternoon, and descending into the evening and nighttime. And at the bottom of the breath where there is nothing to be done but simply to wait and rest, waiting until the next dawn of the breath arises and so on with every cycle of breath, effortlessly noticing the cycle of the breath unfolding... And with increasing spaciousness and ease, the body settles deeper into stillness.

Welcoming Creativity

And in the space of awareness that is Yoga Nidra, invite your attention to travel down on the exhalation as if coming to the space behind the center of the breast bone, as if the exhalation could carry your awareness inside to the space of the heart, exhaling into the heart-space. And simply to be there in that space, at the end of the exhalation, to invite that space to be a place of welcome for whatever creative insight may be arising now or in the future.

To rest the awareness in that space of the heart, and maybe, if it feels appropriate and comfortable to you, to bring a little question, a question about the next step in whatever creative project you may be involved with, whatever the next step might be, maybe bring a question there about that step, but it's simply enough to rest the awareness in the space of the heart, and to know that there is a welcome space...

Rotation of Consciousness with Nyasa

And from that space now, from the end of the next exhalation, invite for the experience of the whole body to be as the night sky, at the end of the exhalation, settling into the nighttime of the breath, and inviting this experience of the whole body to be as a beautiful, dark night sky...

And as the awareness travels around the night sky of the body, it's as if little stars shine in the night sky of the body, as if the whole body becomes filled with constellations of shining stars in the night sky of the body.

Begin by inviting the awareness to travel to the crown of the head as if a little star was shining there. And then allow for the awareness to travel down to the space between the two eyebrows, a star there. And then down between the two collarbones, in the space of the hollow of the base of the throat, a little star shining there. And then stars shining on the right arm from the right shoulder, elbow, wrist, the tip of the right hand's thumb, index finger, middle finger, ring finger, and little finger. Stars in the space of the right wrist, elbow, and shoulder.

Invite the awareness to settle back at the star between the collarbones and then across and over to a star placed in the left shoulder, elbow, and wrist. More stars at the left hand's thumb, index finger, middle finger, ring finger, and little finger. A star in the space of the left wrist, elbow, and shoulder.

And back to the hollow at the base of the throat, a star between the collarbones. A star down in the space, behind the place, at the center behind the breastbone. A star behind the left breast, back to the star at the center of the breastbone, a star behind the right breast, and back to the star behind the center of the breastbone. And all the way down, a star in the belly, behind the navel. A star in the pelvis. Let there be a star in the center of the pelvis.

And then over to the right hip, knee, ankle, and five little stars, one each on the tip of the right big toe, second toe, third toe, fourth toe, and fifth toe. A star inside the right ankle, knee, and hip. Back to the star in the pelvis, over to the left hip, knee, ankle, and five little stars at the tips of the left big toe, second toe, third toe, fourth toe, and fifth toe. A star inside the left ankle, knee, and hip.

Back to the star in the pelvis, up to the star behind the navel, and up to the star behind the center of the breastbone. And up to the star between the collarbones, to the star between the eyebrows, and to the star on the crown of the head.

And in the space of awareness, which is Yoga Nidra, be aware of the whole body resting with a constellation of shining stars in the night sky of the body as the body rests.

And in that space of awareness, invite for the attention to rest now, into the place, behind the space, between the two eyebrows, the star there. Invite for the awareness to settle now, into the place, at the space, between the two collarbones, the star there.

And then come home to the deep heart's core. To the space, behind the center of the breastbone, to the star there. A tiny star in that space.

Welcome home to yourself. And now in the space of awareness, which is Yoga Nidra, let the incoming breath make spaces between all of the stars in the great constellation of the night sky of the body. As if when the breath comes in, a little more space opens up between each star and its neighbor. Maybe as the breath comes in, the stars move out, wide across the great expanse of the heavens, and then as the breath goes out, it's as if all those stars from up there in the heavens very gently settle down into the earth of the body. And with every breath that comes in, the constellation of those stars in the night sky of the body would open out a little wider and bigger. And with every breath that goes out, all of those stars in the constellation of the night sky of the body would settle down into the earth of the body so gently, as if at the end of every exhalation, each star would find a little home for its brightness, in the earth of the body.

So gentle and soft. So bright. Each breath in, the stars spread out a little wider, a little higher, and each breath out, all the brightness of all of those stars lands gently in the earth of the body.

And be with these two forms of awareness for the next few rounds of breath... Spaciousness on the inhale as the stars spread out. Welcoming the brightness of the stars to land in the body as the breath settles. As the breath comes in, all the stars spread out a little, and as the breath goes out, the brightness of the stars lands in the body gently.

Expanding Awareness

And invite the possibility that both those forms of awareness could be present at the same time. So how would that be? ... In the space of awareness, which is Yoga Nidra, to welcome in the spaciousness that comes in with the inhale, and at the same time welcoming in this sense of grounding the light of the stars, as if there could be spaciousness, expansiveness, and grounded-ness, fully earthed at the same time. So how would that be? To be expansive yet fully grounded at the same time...

And let go of that exploration, and now simply invite the light of all of the stars in the constellation of the body to simply settle into the space behind the center of the breastbone. As if when the breath goes out, all the light of all the stars would shine in behind the space at the center of the breastbone.

And then, from that tiny bright light, the heart center, when the breath comes in, to allow for all of the stars to spread out wide and high amongst the heavens, and when the breath leaves for all of the light of all of those stars to gather into the center of the heart, at the back of the space, behind the center of the breastbone.

So moving between those two forms of awareness, a great expansiveness on the inhale with space between the stars, and then gathering in on the exhale all the light of all of those stars, settling right in behind the center of the breastbone, into the space of the deep heart's core. Moving between those two forms of awareness with each round of breath.

And then in the space of awareness, which is Yoga Nidra, invite for those two forms of awareness to coexist. So how would it be, at the same time, to have that expansiveness but to be fully centered at a single point of focus—to have that centered single point of focus, but yet to be in a space of expansiveness at the same time. So how would that be?... Where would that be?...

Sensing Creative Awareness

And then letting go of that exploration, coming in with the awareness, settled in the deep heart's core, behind the center of the middle of the breastbone, come home to yourself and simply be in the space of the heart...

And in that space, feel that there is a welcome for the awareness to come home and for whatever creative insight might be just right, just now. Perhaps for that to be present, for there to be an answer to the question that you may have had at the beginning of the practice. But it is more than enough to simply rest the awareness in this space. (Pause.)

Reawakening and Closing

Feeling into the warm welcome that's in the space of the heart, breathe a little louder, and sense now that the warm welcome could be extended out as you breathe and begin moving and stretching... Stretching your arms, legs, and more. (Pause.)

As we come toward the end of this practice of Yoga Nidra, that you could carry a warm welcome for all that arises in the rest of your day and for all that unfolds in the dreams of the night. Breathing freely and easily a little louder now.

Reawakening as you come to the end of this practice of Yoga Nidra for creativity. When you're ready, roll to your side for as long as you like, and then rise up to sitting. Thank you.

Uma Dinsmore-Tuli is a mother, Yoga therapist, teacher-trainer and retreat leader. Her knowledgeable yet intimate approach has made her one of Europe's most sought-after teachers. Her PhD is in communications and her diploma in Yoga therapy is from the Yoga Biomedical Trust. Uma is cofounder of the Yoga Nidra Network and has developed

Total Yoga Nidra and Nidra Shakti. She has special expertise in women's health and Yoga Nidra. She lives in Stroud, UK. Visit YogaNidraNetwork.org for more.

References and Resources

Websites

YogaNidraNetwork.org

Umadinsmoretuli.com

Books and Audios

Nidra Shakti: An Encyclopaedia of Yoga Nidra. Stroud, UK. Sitaram and Sons, 2021.

Heartfelt Yoga Nidra Meditation

Julie Lusk

Time: 30 minutes

Summary: A heartfelt Yoga Nidra experience is guided for awakening compassion, inner knowing, and unconditional peace. The process includes mindbody sensing based on maps of the sensory-motor cortex, chakras, and marma points. Sohum, the natural sound of the breath is used as a mantra. Sohum is translated as, "I am That" in the Vedas, an ancient yogic text. It helps us feel interconnected with and supported by Universal energy. Inner eye gazing (chidakasha) further calms the mind while wakening intuition and is a prelude to heartfelt imagery and inner guidance. Ample time is given for dwelling in the peaceful spaciousness of Yoga Nidra.

Additional Notes: The mindbody sensing, sohum breathing, and the inner eye gazing segments can all be used on their own to reap their benefits.

Stages	Process / Techniques
Preparation and settling in	Savasana
Sankalpa	Heartfelt pledge
Physical: Anna-maya kosha	Mindbody sensing with rotation of consciousness
Energetic: Prana-maya kosha	Sohum mantra breathing
Mental: Mano-maya kosha	Inner eye gazing (chidakasha)
Intuitive: Vijnana-maya kosha	Intuitive knowing with heart-centered imagery
Bliss: Ananda-maya kosha	Heart-centered imagery
True Self: Atman	True nature awareness

Stages	Process / Techniques
Sankalpa	Heartfelt pledge
Reawakening and closing	

Preparation and Settling In

It's time for Yoga Nidra. Please settle yourself in comfortably, lying fully supported in savasana and using props to your advantage. Comfort is key to prevent physical distractions right from the start. To enable you to be as still as possible, you may like a thin pillow under your head or to support your neck, an eye pillow, a firm cushion or blanket under your knees or thighs, and something to cover up with to stay warm. Know that you can make personal, mindful adjustments as needed. Vaguely hearing what's going on is common, especially when you're engaged with the Yoga Nidra experience. Even still, use my voice as an anchor to the present moment. Feel free to go along with as much or as little as you like. Please take a minute for adding your own reminders in support of having a good experience and to remind yourself to listen, participate, stay alert, and accept what happens. *(Pause about 10 seconds.)*

Let's begin. Take a big breath in through your nose and sigh it out... Next, with eyes closed, start lifting and lowering your eyebrows several times... and allow them to rest in stillness... Begin moving your jaw all around, releasing lots of tension... Rest your jaw, feeling tightness and tension draining away, perhaps feeling a softness all around your jaw and mouth... Begin rolling your head from side to side... and bringing it back to the center. Have your nose, chest, and navel in a straight line. Feel free to have your chin tucked slightly to open up airflow... Take a big breath in and sigh it out... You can take several sighing breaths on your own. *(Pause.)*

Scoot your shoulders down from your ears and snuggle your shoulder blades nicely underneath for comfort... Place your arms beside you and a comfortable distance away from your body... To relax your hands, stretch your fingers all about... open and close them a few times... For now, allow your fingers to rest comfortably with your palms up.

Start noticing your low back... Adjust under there until it feels more stable and even... Begin wiggling your toes... and rest... Have your feet a comfortable distance apart or have them on the floor with your knees up or propped... Scan your body, picking up on what's happening...and make your own adjustments for even more comfort and ease. *(Pause.)*

Heartfelt Pledge

It's time for your heartfelt pledge—a wise intention that comes from deep inside that warms your heart for developing a positive quality like confidence or loving kindness, or for changing a behavior, supporting spirituality, or reflecting something that gives meaning and purpose to your life's direction—your sankalpa. Consistency pays off, so use the one that you've established, giving it time to take root, grow, and thrive. If you have one, repeat yours silently about three times, with heartfelt conviction.

Otherwise, this could be the time to formulate one. Let one come to you. There's no pressure. When it does, keep it positive, clear, brief, and sincere. Say it to yourself in the present tense as if it's already happened. *(Pause.)*

Sense what it'd be like if your heartfelt pledge were already happening. Exploring how it would look...what it would feel like...and the type of actions or behaviors involved...using your imagination to get into it. *(Pause.)* Take a big breath in and sigh it out, letting it all go. *(Pause.)*

If you'd like to make any adjustments for more comfort, feel free to do it now. *(Pause.)* Please remind yourself to stay aware and alert instead of sleeping.

MindBody Sensing with Rotation of Consciousness

Let's take an awareness tour throughout your body. Simply follow along, flowing as we go. If it helps, it's fine to picture these places, experience physical sensations, or have a concept of it, going with whatever comes easiest. You may silently repeat each location to yourself as you mentally follow along for experiencing the flowing of energy. There's no need for any movements. In fact, it's better if you can stay still. If your attention wanders needlessly, just pick back up wherever we are.

Taking your attention down to your right foot...and noticing your big toe...second toe...third toe...fourth toe...and baby toe...Sensing the top of the foot...bottom of the foot...heel...ankle...calf...knee...thigh...hip...Going up the side of the body to the armpit...shoulder...elbow...wrist...the thumb...index finger...middle finger...ring finger...and little finger...back of the hand ... palm ... And now the whole hand ... whole arm ... whole shoulder ... whole right side ... whole hip ... whole leg ... and the whole right foot.

And over to the left foot ... the big toe ... second toe ... third toe ... fourth toe ... and baby toe ... Top of the foot ... bottom of the foot ... heel ... ankle ... calf ... knee ... thigh ... hip ... Going up the side of the body to the armpit ... shoulder ... elbow ... wrist ... the thumb ... index finger ... middle finger ... ring finger ... and little finger ... back of hand ... palm ... Now the whole hand ... whole arm ... whole shoulder ... whole left side ... whole hip ... whole leg ... and the whole left foot.

Noticing both feet ... both legs ... the base of the spine ... low back ... mid-back ... upper back ... neck ... back of the head ... top of the head ... the forehead ... right eyebrow ... left eyebrow ... space between the eyebrows ... right eyelid ... left eyelid ... right eyeball ... left eyeball ... both eyes, sensing both eyes ... and the line between the eyelids, where the eyelids touch. *(Pause.)*

The bridge of the nose ... tip of the nose ... upper lip ... lower lip ... moisten your lips if you like ... Jaw ... Right ear ... over the top of the head to the left ear ... and inside the head between the ears, the inside center point between the ears ... Inside the mouth ... roof of the mouth ... bottom of the mouth ... inside cheeks ... and sensing your tongue and where it is ... perhaps using your tongue to tickle the roof of your mouth or run it around in there ... and allowing the tongue to softly hover in there, quietly ... and sensing the moisture, feeling the moisture inside the mouth ...

Feel free to swallow or clear your throat if you wish ... settling further into comfort and ease ... Noticing the throat ... base of the throat between the collarbones ... Sensing, getting in touch with the heart ... the upper abdomen ... navel ... lower abdomen ... base of the spine.

And the whole back side ... including the heels, head, hands ... and being in touch with all the contact points where the back of your body touches the surface supporting you ... and noticing how the surface totally supports you ... And all the contact points at once ... And the whole front side ... and the space around your front side ... and now both sides, front and back as one ... And noticing the head ... face ... brain ... and the head, face, and brain, all as one ... Sensing and noticing the whole self, the entire self ... and inside your whole self ... Sensing into the space surrounding your whole self ... And sensing both inside and around your whole self... your whole self... your whole self as one-ness. *(Pause about 10 seconds.)*

Sohum Mantra Breathing

Readjust for comfort, if needed, so you're nice and comfortable... And settling in even better, remembering to stay aware and alert while noticing your entire experience...

Turning your attention to your breathing for a while... Leave it be. There's no need to fix or change it. *(Pause.)* Feel free to rest your attention around the home of your heart while you're breathing... as if your heart is breathing... being centered with your heart... at home with your heart. *(Pause.)*

Now, begin using "sohum" as a mantra. Use it as a relaxing lullaby and for staying awake with awareness. Here's how. Each time you inhale, silently say, "so." Each time you exhale, silently say, "hum." That's it. Repeating "so" when breathing in and "hum" when breathing out. As soon as you notice your mind has wandered, kindly and gently turn your attention back to breathing with "sohum." *(Pause about 1 minute.)*

Continuing on, you may simply listen to your breath, noticing how the inhalation naturally sounds like "so" on its own and how the exhalation sounds like "hum." Practicing awareness without words. Whenever it helps, feel free to silently say "sohum." *(Pause about 1 minute.)*

Inner Eye Gazing (Chidakasha)

Allowing your tongue to soften, hovering in the mouth, and simultaneously having your breathing heart-centered... Start focusing attention on your eyes, becoming aware of your eyes, cradled, and resting in their sockets...

If you'd like to go deeper, become aware of the eyelids touching and covering your eyes, like eyeshades. Even though your eyes are closed, you can still see. Start focusing your inner vision, watching whatever appears on the inside shade of your eyelids. It might appear dark, there may be some color, perhaps some shapes, coming and going... It doesn't matter what's there—what matters is watching whatever comes and goes... There's no need for making comments about it, refocusing whenever distractions happen... Let your eyes rest even more now and become quiet, yet still watching the inner space... simply looking and softly gazing and watching in stillness. *(Pause about 1 minute.)*

Intuitive Knowing with Heart-Centered Imagery

And having your attention with your heart center and your breathing... Quiet eyes... Soft tongue... Feeling heart-centered, more and more.

Take your attention to whatever you're experiencing now. Perhaps it's a sense of inner peace, of truth, of delight, of deep satisfaction, and allowing its Presence. *(Pause.)*

If it helps, remember a time when your heart felt full. Free. Perhaps you were in nature, mesmerized by a beautiful sunset. Perhaps having a good time with others, laughing and loving. Or maybe cuddling with a pet. Bringing something alive, real or imagined, that touches your heart... Sensing it by having a concept of what it looked like... how it felt... sounded, tasted, and smelled... Embellishing this heartfelt feeling, however you like, bringing it alive... and feeling what it was like all over again. The physical feelings... the emotional feelings... all the heartfelt feelings...

And, if you like, let the memory fade away... not having to rely on anything else for heartfelt awareness of contentment, joyfulness, and ease. Being in touch with this constant, unconditional inner joy that is already yours, always. *(Pause.)*

And it's a portal to your heart, deeply knowing your heart as loving and lovable. *(Pause about 10 seconds.)* Centered with your heart... quiet eyes... soft tongue... heart-centered... And your heart is like an antenna, transmitting qualities of the heart, capable of giving and receiving genuine, heartfelt love. *(Pause.)* And listening with your heart for guidance. *(Pause about 1 minute.)*

True Nature Awareness

And letting all this fade away into blissful, timeless, spacious awareness of unconditional love, peace, joy, and Presence. *(Pause 2–4 minutes.)*

Heartfelt Pledge

It's time to transition, flowing into remembering your heartfelt pledge. Bringing your sankalpa back to mind to repeat three or so times with feeling, and from your heart, allowing it to sink in deeply and meaningfully. *(Pause.)*

Imagine how it would be if it were already so. *(Pause about 15 seconds.)* And so it is... Take a big breath in... and sigh it out.

Reawakening and Closing

It's time to start coming back with full awareness and wakefulness, and to bring back with you all the benefits of Yoga Nidra to benefit yourself as well as others.

Become aware of your breathing, following its coming and going. Listening to its sounds of "so" upon inhalation and "hum" upon exhalation... It's good to breathe more fully for a while, allowing the deeper breath to bring about awakening... experiencing mental clarity, like a brilliant sunrise... Now you're becoming more aware of the whole body, simply being here, experiencing peaceful, comforting, and joyful energy. *(Pause.)*

Becoming awake and aware of this time and place... You're becoming very clear-headed and so wide awake and noticing the feeling of being totally relaxed and refreshed.

Become increasingly more aware of your Presence in these surroundings, of belonging... Sensing what's above... what's all around... and sensing what's below... Getting a direct experience of being present in this room, here and now.

When you're ready, begin moving your body, stretching it however you wish. *(Pause for stretching.)* It's time to get ready to roll over onto your side... Okay now, roll over and curl up for a while and eventually sit in a comfortable position. *(Pause.)*

Rest your hands on your lap. Touch the tips of your thumbs and index fingers together. Soak it in. *(Pause.)* When you're ready, blink your eyes open, blending the inner and outer worlds together as one... Inhale deeply and let it go... Notice whatever you notice. *(Pause.)*

Remembering to follow your heart's truth and its guidance for living a life of meaning and purpose. Sohum breathing can be used anytime you like.

Peace, peace, peace. (Om shanti, shanti, shanti.)

Tender Time Yoga Nidra

Julie Lusk

Time: 30 minutes

Summary: This gently and effectively eases you into deeper stages of relaxation to an uplifting, deeply felt sense of peacefulness. It begins with a wonderful variation of progressive muscle relaxation (PMR). A light amount of tension is used instead of tensing muscle groups to their maximum. This technique enables you to develop sensitivity to low levels of tension that often go unnoticed. It is effective when full muscle tension is contraindicated or when you're interested in trying something different. The booster breath is used by adding a pause and an extra boost after inhaling and exhaling. Mindfulness and guided imagination practice lead into feeling peaceful, spacious, and timeless. Intuition and unconditional joy often result.

Stages	Process / Techniques
Preparation and settling in	Savasana
Sankalpa	Heartfelt pledge
Physical: Anna-maya kosha	Tender time relaxation: Progressive muscle relaxation with light tension
Energetic: Prana-maya kosha	Booster breath
Mental: Mano-maya kosha	Mindful guided imagination for mental and emotional clearing
Intuitive: Vijnana-maya kosha	Insightful awareness
Bliss: Ananda-maya kosha	Joyful rest
True Self: Atman	Pure awareness

Stages	Process / Techniques
Sankalpa	Heartfelt pledge
Reawakening and closing	

Preparation and Settling In

Lie down on your back or sit in a chair. Settle yourself in for maximum comfort and ease. With your eyes closed, lift and lower your eyebrows a few times... now, let them smooth out and be still... Next, move your mouth all around, stretching and moving your lips and jaw... let your mouth rest... Slowly roll your head from side to side a couple of times... bring it to rest so the center of your chin is aligned with your chest and navel... Have the very back of your head directly on the floor or thin pillow with your chin tucked slightly toward your throat... Move your shoulders down from your ears and tuck your shoulder blades in comfortably... Next, open and close your hands and stretch your fingers... let them become still, with your palms up... Start noticing your low back, hips, and buttocks... Lift up there and settle back down, fuss around under there until it feels as comfortable and supported as possible, using props as needed... Take your attention down to your toes and stretch them... and rest... To release tension in your legs and back, place your feet twelve to twenty-four inches apart... Take a moment to notice what's happening and then make your own adjustments... Feel free to smooth out your clothes or props... It's time to settle in for this Yoga Nidra experience. *(Pause.)*

Heartfelt Pledge

If you have one, feel free to begin saying your sankalpa, your own resolve. Otherwise, you're invited to welcome one in if you wish. It's a positive, concise statement that's said like it is already true. A heartfelt pledge to support your life's meaning and purpose or foster a helpful quality or characteristic that's personal to you. Examples are, "I have abundance," "My life is unfolding in harmonious ways," or "I am patient, more and more." It's okay if nothing comes or this doesn't appeal to you now. *(Pause.)*

Tender Time Relaxation

It's fine to adjust your position and clothing for maximum comfort and ease... Settling yourself in, more and more... Please bring your attention to your right foot... begin bringing a light amount of tension to your toes and foot, just until you start feeling it... Hold it... notice... and let it all go, softening like butter, melting away... Now, take your attention to your leg and start tensing it ever so tenderly... hold it... notice... and let the tension dissolve, all at once... Let's go on to the left side... Please bring your attention to your left foot... begin bringing a light amount of tension to your toes and foot, just until you start feeling it... notice... and let it all go, melting like ice in hot water... Now, take your attention to your leg and start tenderly tensing it ever so slightly... notice... and let the tension dissolve, all at once... Both your legs and feet are feeling more at ease as tension leaves more and more. *(Pause.)* Notice how easy it is to tense and relax.

Now for the upper body. Bring your awareness to your dominant hand... When you're ready, start to squeeze your hand as little as you can, just until you start noticing it... study it... Now, let go to relax your fingers and hand... feeling the difference... Let's do the same for that arm by bringing a tender amount of pressure to it... hold it... notice... and completely let go, allowing your arm and hand to relax softly, more and more... Focusing on your other hand now, create a tiny bit of tension in your fingers and hand, just for now... notice ... and let it all dissolve... noticing the difference... And moving your awareness up your arm... start making a little amount of pressure, the minimum amount needed to notice it... notice... now let it leave, more and more... Please go back to your dominant side... This time simply pretend to squeeze tension and pressure into it... notice... and let it totally evaporate like fog lifting... noticing what happens. Noticing how your imagination effects your body. *(Pause.)*

Know that your body can become even more relaxed. If you wish, take your awareness to your buttocks and belly... Bring a slight amount of tension to these areas, just until you barely feel it... notice... and let go, feeling the softening, and how your body feels like it's pressing firmly into the surface supporting it. Let this happen.

Please notice your heart and lungs... Slowly breathe in, sensing this area filling up, feeling your lungs expanding and notice all the sensations involved ... notice... and let all the air out... Once again, breathe in, filling up and sensing, feeling the expansion in your chest, heart, sides, and back...notice...and let all the air out...Notice if your level of relaxation is growing. *(Pause.)*

It's time for your face, noticing the sensations that are happening throughout your face...Please press your lips together, ever so slightly...notice it...and let go, allowing your lips to soften and relax...Go ahead and press your tongue against the roof of your mouth or the back of your teeth...notice it...and let go so your tongue can hover quietly in there...Feel free to press again and then release even more...relaxing more and more...Slightly scrunch up your eyes and forehead, just so it's noticeable...notice...and let it smooth out, nice and even...One more time, bringing a tiny bit of tension and pressure to your whole face...notice it...and let go...becoming more and more aware of the changing sensations of tension and relaxation. *(Pause.)* Knowing that you have ways to exchange tension for relaxation.

Please use your mind's eye to scan your body, noticing all the sensations present, noticing textures, just as they are...It's your choice to continue your observations or to use this technique or another one to add to your experience. *(Pause.)*

Remember, this is your time to explore and notice feeling deeply relaxed while staying alert, no sleeping...If needed, feel free to adjust your position and then settle back in. *(Pause.)*

Booster Breath

If you like, you can linger where you are or use your breath to relax further by smoothing out any static, allowing you to sink into relaxation further.

Take your attention to your breath, following its movements of naturally inhaling and exhaling through your nose for the next few rounds of breathing...Each time your attention drifts off, gently bring it back to your breathing. It's good practice to catch your mind wandering and gently returning it to your breathing. There's no need to do anything else, just follow a few more rounds of your breath, just for now. *(Pause.)*

Would you like to use your breath to focus your awareness even more and for becoming more relaxed?...If so, listen first and then follow along. At the top of each inhalation, pause and sip a little more air in and then breathe out naturally. Okay now, each time you breathe in, pause, breathe in a little extra, and then let the air naturally leave. Continue boosting each inhalation with a little more air and an easy-going exhalation...Take your time. Noticing what this is like, topping each inhalation off, time after time. *(Pause.)* Let your breathing return to its natural ways, simply breathing in and out naturally, noticing what you notice. *(Pause.)*

It's time to shift your focus to your exhalations. Listen first and then follow along. At the bottom of each exhalation, pause and exhale a bit more, letting the next inhalation come on its own. Okay now, each time you breathe out, pause, send a little more out, then naturally breathe back in. Over and over again, breathing a little extra out at the bottom of your exhalations...Take your time. Noticing what this is like, breathing out a little extra after each exhalation, again and again. *(Pause.)* Let your breathing return to its natural ways, simply breathing in and out naturally, noticing what you notice. *(Pause.)*

It's time to do this with both the inhalations and exhalations...It's like putting a bookend or an exclamation point on both sides of each inhalation and exhalation. Take your time. When you're ready, feel yourself breathing in...pause a second...boost it with a little extra air, and start breathing out. At the end of your exhalation, pause a second...and send a bit more out...continuing to add a little more air at one end and subtracting more at the other end...Continue with this for the next few minutes. Remember to gently bring your attention back to your breathing each time you get unnecessarily distracted. *(Pause 1 minute or more.)*

It's time to let go of this and let your breathing become effortless, naturally coming and going on its own...Noticing what you notice. *(Pause.)*

Mindful Guided Imagination for Mental and Emotional Clearing

Please continue following the movement or feel of each breath as it comes and goes. Let it be just as it is...Notice if there's an urge to change it or form an opinion about it. It's okay, be curious and interested...Notice this when it happens, and return your attention to your natural breathing, in and out. *(Pause.)*

Your breath may start reminding you of the wind blowing outside, like how the wind comes and goes...Sometimes it's a gentle breeze, other times it's gusty, and sometimes it's quite strong...Imagine being outside, feeling the wind blow...imagine it blowing through the trees...watch it rustling the leaves...

listening to its sound... scents carried by the wind... fascinated by the wind. *(Pause.)*

Now move your attention to your thoughts and feelings and how they're like the wind. Sometimes gentle, sometimes fierce. Sometimes noticeable, sometimes not. How thoughts and feelings are like leaves blowing in the wind... and becoming more aware of what's on your mind... letting thoughts and feelings come and go, like leaves blowing in the wind... There's no need to name them, or even prefer one over another, simply noticing your thoughts and feelings, just for now... making room for whatever is occurring, as it comes and goes. *(Pause.)*

Watching them as they pass on by, allowing thoughts and feelings to move on by, taking flight with the wind... impartially observing any thoughts and feelings as they appear... There's no point in getting involved in what they are, but just notice them, like leaves blowing. *(Pause.)* If you doubt yourself, wondering if you're doing this right, it's just another thought. Toss it like a leaf into the wind to go away... If you're feeling bored or maybe think this isn't for you, it's just another thought to give to the wind... Feel free to watch the leaves being tossed by the wind... a gust of wind comes to clear away outdated thoughts, feelings, and limiting beliefs, blowing away and clearing out what's no longer needed. *(Pause.)*

Let your heart fly like the wind... Fly your way home.

And the wind begins to become still... and the leaves begin to settle into the quietude. *(Pause.)*

How about being aware of the vast and open sky itself... Where the wind blows, causing clouds to take shape and change again and again... and how thoughts and feelings are like clouds, forming and evaporating, just like clouds in the sky. *(Pause.)*

Insightful Awareness with Joyful Rest and Pure Awareness

And waking up the dimension of yourself that's like the sky, vast and open ... allowing and including thoughts, feelings, and everything else to come and go, like leaves and clouds blowing about in the vast sky... It's awareness itself, always present and always awake. Sinking into it during this quiet pause. *(Pause 1 minute or more.)*

And imagining the clouds clearing, the winds settling down...and as this happens, there's open space, timeless space, as vast and infinite as the sky...It's awareness itself, it's that part of you that is always present and always awake. That makes space for insights, unconditional peace, and joy to be present during this quiet pause. *(Pause 1 minute or more.)*

Heartfelt Pledge

This is the time for your sankalpa to appear, your heartfelt pledge to support a life of meaning, perhaps a positive quality...Letting it float into your awareness, taking shape, more and more...Perhaps it appears as a word or phrase or an image...perhaps it's formless...perhaps letting it ring through you from your heart and soul...imagining how it looks and sounds and feels...allowing it to take shape in your life, more and more. *(Pause.)*

Reawakening and Closing

It's time to transition back, bringing with you all the insights and understandings you've received, for your sake, and for the sake of others. So, with this greater awareness of yourself, begin breathing more deeply, feeling the breath beginning to awaken you...feeling your breath coming and going, like the wind...

It's time to stretch your body in ways that come naturally, moving your arms and legs and moving everything else...Notice the movements, the physical sensations as you're stretching. *(Pause.)*

If you're lying down, please roll to your side and curl up...Eventually, use your arms for support to press yourself up to sitting. *(Pause.)* Rest your hands on your lap...To seal this in and for maintaining the connection, touch the tips of the thumbs to the index fingers. *(Pause.)*

Open your eyes and let your vision come alive. Glance around, fully aware of what's before you and how it looks. Soak in the shapes, colors, textures, and your surroundings...looking for something that is blue...gazing at the smallest thing you can find...Being aware of sounds...being aware. *(Pause.)* Begin stretching about, awakening more and more.

Peace, peace, peace. (Om shanti, shanti, shanti.)

Chair Yoga Nidra

Julie Lusk

Time: 20 minutes

Summary: Practicing in a chair is a nice change and a good option when it is inconvenient or uncomfortable to lie down. Afterall, it is important to have Yoga Nidra skills in a variety of positions and settings.

Systematic stretching for tension release is practiced throughout your body. Focused breathing is used for increasing inner stability and to improve concentration. Mindfulness awakens inner knowing and unconditional peace and joy. A hand gesture, called the sankalpa mudra, is used to empower your heartfelt pledge (sankalpa). Mudras are like Yoga postures done with your hands that can be used anytime. They can have positive effects on your body, mind, and spirit, and enliven your life force and energy. There are hundreds of them.

Use a comfortable high-backed chair to support your head, neck, and shoulders. A neck pillow travelers use can support your head. Otherwise, put the chair against a wall with a cushion between your head and the wall. To help relieve back tension, put something like a block, book, or pillow under your feet so they are flat on the floor. Make sure there is enough room for stretching your arms and legs straight out in front of you.

Stages	Process / Techniques
Preparation and settling in	Savasana
Sankalpa	Heartfelt pledge with the sankalpa mudra, a hand gesture
Physical: Anna-maya kosha	Systematic stretching and tension release

Stages	Process / Techniques
Energetic: Prana-maya kosha	Focused breathing
Mental: Mano-maya kosha	Mindfulness
Intuitive: Vijnana-maya kosha	Insights and inner knowing
Bliss: Ananda-maya kosha	Sensing inner peace
True Self: Atman	True nature awareness
Sankalpa	Heartfelt pledge
Reawakening and closing	

Preparation and Settling In

Sit down in a chair. Place your feet firmly on the floor to relieve low back strain. It's best for your head, chin, and chest to be aligned. Do not cross your legs, feet, or arms for better circulation. Close your eyes or have them slightly open.

Heartfelt Pledge

Let's begin. Take a big breath in and sigh it out... Go ahead and do this a few more times on your own. *(Pause.)*

Rest your left hand on your right thigh with your palm facing up. Softly, cup your right palm crossed over the left one with a little room between your palms and creating a space for your heartfelt pledge to naturally incubate, take root, and grow. This hand gesture (mudra) will energize and empower your intention. Allow your breathing to flow for a few rounds, being mindful of your experience.

You're welcome to start by remembering your heartfelt pledge. If you have one, repeat it three or so times, remembering to be consistent, positive, brief, and in the present tense, like it's happening right now.

Or, perhaps, let something arise from within you, a quality that supports your highest good and life direction... It's okay if nothing seems to be happening. Trust that it will when the time is right. Or, for now, you can silently say something like, "I am getting healthier, more and more" or "My true nature is peace." If this doesn't appeal to you, just skip it.

Take a big breath in and sigh it out while un-cupping your hands. Rest them on your lap.

Systematic Stretching and Tension Release

It's time to relax by moving or tensing each part of your body and then drain the tightness away by letting go. Skip anything that's inappropriate for you. During relaxation, it's typical for your muscles to soften and feel warmer, heavier, quieter, and comfortable, so let that happen. Your breath is likely to even out.

It's time to lean into the chair back, sensing the contact points between you and the chair, noticing how it's supporting you ... and feeling your legs being supported by the chair seat. Your arms can rest on your lap and have both feet on the floor. Let's work from the ground up.

To relax your *feet*, lift them up and start circling your ankles for three or four times ... and circle them in the other direction three or four times ... Put your feet back on the floor.

To relax your *lower legs*, hold your legs straight out ... gently but firmly, point your toes away from you to stretch them, feeling the tension in your legs, especially in your ankles and shins ... let your feet fall back to the floor ... Notice if you're feeling the sensation of quieting into relaxation yet.

To relax your lower legs more, hold both legs straight out again and point your toes back toward your head, focusing on your calves ... Let your feet fall back to the floor ... Let go and relax.

To relax your *upper legs*, press your knees and thighs together and hold ... Notice the tension in your upper legs ... Let go and relax, letting your legs rest a comfortable distance apart.

Notice how you're feeling more and more at ease. Perhaps your legs are feeling heavy, warm, and relaxed ... Resolve to keep them still and relaxed for now. Sinking into the chair, more and more.

To relax your *abdomen*, pull in your abdominal muscles as much as you want and hold ... Notice the compressed feeling ... Let go, soften, and relax, feeling and allowing all the knots inside loosening. *(Pause.)*

Now push your abdomen outward as much as you like, feeling your abdominal wall expand, making room for all your internal organs and giving them space ... Let go, soften, and relax ... allowing this area to soften further.

Still focusing on your *belly*, take a deep breath into the bottom of your lungs and hold... and let it rush out.

To relax your *chest*, take a deep breath into your upper lungs and hold... Let the air rush out.

Take another full, deep breath in, filling your *lungs* up completely and hold it... Let all the air rush out, feeling more and more at ease.

Notice feeling a full, gentle inflation when inhaling and a gentle deflation when exhaling. Go ahead and notice this movement for a couple rounds of breathing. Each time your focus wanders, bring it back to breathing... It's okay to feel yourself relaxing even more each time you breathe out. *(Pause.)*

To relax your *shoulders*, breathe in while pressing your shoulders up toward your ears and hold... Now, drop your shoulders while releasing your breath... Let's repeat. Breathe in lots of fresh air while pressing your shoulders up toward your ears and hold... Now, drop your shoulders, releasing your breath.

To relax your *upper arms and biceps*, bring your hands up to your shoulders and tense your biceps and hold... noticing the tension in your upper arms... let your arms fall to your lap and relax... Notice how your arms are feeling warm, heavy, and comfortable, more and more.

To relax your *lower arms*, hold your arms straight out in front of you with your palms facing down. Bend your wrists so your fingers point toward the ceiling and hold, feeling the tension in your forearms... drop your hands to your lap and relax... Notice the feeling of comfort in your arms, perhaps warm and cozy.

To relax your *hands*, make a fist and hold tightly... now spread your fingers apart and hold... Let go and relax, allowing your fingers to uncurl and soften into stillness, more and more... Let your hands and arms relax completely, resting on your lap.

It's time to relax your *neck*. Tip your head over to the right side, moving your ear toward your right shoulder. Be careful not to strain... Come back to the middle... Now tip your head toward your left shoulder and feel the sensations... Bring your head back up to center. Let it wobble until it comes to a comfortable resting position.

To relax the front of your neck, bring your chin toward your chest and hold... Lift your head up and relax. Let your head wobble until comfortable and balanced.

To release *jaw* tension, open your mouth and move your jaw up and down and sideways, working out all tension... Relax and let your teeth part slightly.

To relax your *mouth* even more, press your lips together tightly... Let go and relax, softening your lips... Now press your tongue against the roof of your mouth or into the teeth... Let go and relax... Moisten your lips if you like and let your teeth part slightly. Relaxing the tongue can calm down restless thoughts, so let your tongue soften, like it's jelly.

To relax your *nose and cheeks*, wrinkle up your nose and hold... Relax.

To relax your *eyes*, squeeze them tightly together and hold... Relax.

To relax your *forehead*, push your eyebrows down and frown... Relax, letting go... Now lift your eyebrows upward... Let go and relax.

It's time to mentally scan your *entire body*. If you notice any remaining tension, give those areas permission to relax and let go. *(Pause.)*

You're now getting very, very relaxed... Let yourself enjoy this feeling... Allow this feeling to sink in all over.

Focused Breathing

To help settle down restless thoughts and improve concentration, focus on your breathing. Breathing well relaxes your nervous system, specifically when your exhalation is longer than your inhalation.

First, notice the airflow at your nostrils by feeling the air coming in and going out. Keep your attention on your nostrils... noticing the sensations at your nostrils as air comes and goes for several rounds of breathing. *(Pause.)*

Now, begin feeling the air going into your nostrils, down the windpipe, into your lungs, and back out again. Continue breathing gently while following the airflow for three or four breaths. As soon as you notice your focus drifting off, return to gently focusing on flowing air. *(Pause.)*

Mindfulness

Let your focus go, just for now... allowing your breathing to naturally come and go. There's no need to change it at all, simply letting it flow all by itself... feeling it come and go, all by itself. *(Pause about 10 seconds.)*

It's okay to let your attention float for a while... allowing any thoughts, feelings, and sensations to come and go... simply let your attention float on its own. There's no need to get caught up at all, that just gets in your way... Impartially noticing whatever is floating in and out of your awareness. (Pause.) Floating with awareness... aware of a part of you that's curious, an awareness that just lets things happen without having to say anything or do anything about it... making room for whatever is floating, curiously aware, impartially aware. (Pause.)

Insights and Inner Knowing

And allowing ideas and insights to appear, perhaps answers to questions start flowing during this pause. (Pause about 1 minute.) Insights can continue coming afterward and when they're needed.

Sensing Inner Peace

It's fine to go into a place of peace and tranquility... If it helps, imagine a time of feeling at ease. A happy time... a time of feeling content, no matter what. (Pause about 2 minutes.)

True Nature Awareness

And perhaps being surrounded by spaciousness and timelessness. (Pause about 2 minutes.)

Heartfelt Pledge

Once again, place your left hand on your right thigh with your palm up. Cup your right palm crossed over the left palm. It's time to bring your heartfelt pledge up... If you have one, repeat it three or so times.

Or, perhaps, let something arise from within you, a quality that supports your highest good and life direction. (Pause.)

If nothing seems to be happening, trust that it will when the time is right. (Pause.)

Imagine what it would look and feel like for your heartfelt pledge to be happening. (Pause about 1 minute.) Take a big breath in and let it go.

Reawakening and Closing

It's time to start transitioning back to this time and place ... Start to picture or sense the room you're in ... the walls, the ceiling, the floor ... hearing the sounds as they come and go ... sensing the atmosphere ... becoming aware of your Presence in this time and space, right here and now ... hearing the sound of your breath, just for now ... following the sound of your own breath, the life force flowing ...

When you're ready, begin stretching and moving about in ways that feel natural to you ... awakening more and more ... stretching and moving ... bringing back with you the benefits of your practice to help yourself and for the sake of others. And when your eyes open, you'll feel wide awake, alert, and fully aware.

Peace, peace, peace. (Om shanti, shanti, shanti.)

FOUR

Special People and Groups

THESE YOGA NIDRA MEDITATIONS are aimed toward kids, teens, men, women, and military members. Afterall, the approach taken for youngsters will differ from that taken with members of the armed forces and veterans. Please don't limit yourself. We found that adults enjoyed the one for kids, women liked the one aimed for men, etc.

Yoga Nidra for Kids and the Young at Heart–Julie Lusk

The relaxation process used is quite active and incorporates fun guided visualization skills to bring about focus. Imagination is used for sniffing a flower, blowing out a candle, and balloon breathing for diaphragmatic breathing are used. A superhero visits with special messages. Self-soothing skills, memory, and learning abilities are strengthened. Closings for either waking up or sleeping are given.

Yoga Nidra: Conquer Stress for Teen Empowerment–Viviana Collazo

Empowering techniques are used, including breath awareness, sankalpa setting, and a more active method of progressive muscle relaxation (PMR). Self-balancing is done using an imaginary golden substance for clearing tension and increasing vital energy. Self-assurance and an inner connection are nurtured. Hand gestures (mudras) for calming agitation and instilling trust and confidence are taught.

Welcoming Your Well-Rested Woman: A Daring to Rest Yoga Nidra Meditation–Karen Brody

Rotation of consciousness, a touchstone, energy center (chakra) balancing, and soul whispers are used to help women feel supremely relaxed, safe, grounded, creative, and able to take back their power from a rooted place. An invitation to either go to sleep or wake up is given.

Yoga Nidra for Men's Health–Julie Lusk

Progressive muscle relaxation is used to offload stress and regulate the nervous system. Breath control, mental focus, mindfulness, and consulting a team of advisors for insights are used. Options are given for customizing the experience to meet one's own needs.

A Beginning iRest Yoga Nidra Script for Active Duty Service Members, Veterans, Families, Health Care Providers, and Support Staff–Robin Carnes

This script focuses on regulating the autonomic nervous system to help reduce stress-related symptoms. A three-part sankalpa is used to instill safety and meet personal needs. Rotation of consciousness, and sensing, deepening, and counting the breath are used. Welcoming emotions, feelings and thoughts, with opposites and witnessing, allow for an underlying sense of well-being to emerge. The language used is compatible with the military culture.

Yoga Nidra for Kids and the Young at Heart

Julie Lusk

Time: Variable. This script is about 20 minutes. Adjust the time depending on the attention span of the person or group. Use single segments to shorten it. Allow additional time beforehand for instructions and afterward for discussion. Options are given for waking up or going to sleep at the end.

Summary: This enjoyable Yoga Nidra script is perfect for children (and adults). The wording is simple and direct. The process used is more active and incorporates imagination skills to increase attention by keeping the mind busy while relaxation of the body, mind, and spirit happens. Both brain hemispheres are activated during Yoga Nidra. Studies have shown that learning capacity and memory improves, and stress and anxiety are lowered in students by the practice of Yoga Nidra.[21]

Additional Notes: Giggles are good. Afterall, Yoga is all about joyfulness. Goofing off is disruptive. Try "smile-asana." Have everyone repeatedly open and close their mouth a few times, as if it's a door, followed by shutting it, keeping their lips together as if they don't want to let anyone in. Smiling is welcome.

Start slowly by introducing a few stages at a time. Add more as participants become familiar with this exercise and can stay still with their eyes closed for longer periods of time. For example, several breathing techniques are offered. Use all of them or choose fewer depending on the child or group.

As always, feel free to modify this script to make it more effective to your situation and group. For example, it might be necessary to take fewer pauses or repeat the instructions more often than what is written. Keep the pace moving to hold attention. Watch what happens and adjust accordingly.

---

21. Kamakhya Kumar, "Impact on Stress and Anxiety," 405–409.

Stages	Process / Techniques
Preparation and settling in	Playful stretching and savasana
Sankalpa	Heartful pledge for health, happiness, love, good self-esteem, calmness, and focus
Physical: Anna-maya kosha	Lively physical relaxation with active imagination
Energetic: Prana-maya kosha	Options for breath awareness: sniffing and blowing, and breathing slowly and smoothly
Mental: Mano-maya kosha	Superhero visualization
Intuitive: Vijnana-maya kosha	Gifts and messages from superhero
Bliss: Ananda-maya kosha	Guided imagination for happiness and joy
True Self: Atman	Stillness
Sankalpa	Heartfelt pledge for health, happiness, love, good self-esteem, calmness, and focus
Reawakening and closing	Closing for going to sleep or to wake up

Preparation and Settling In

Lie down on your back and stretch your arms and legs out … Wiggle all around. That's right, it's okay to squirm … Stop moving, just for now … let's see how still and quiet you can be, still as a statue and not moving … Put your palms together and quickly rub them up and down … Put your palms over your closed eyes … no peeking … Put your hands by your sides. Please keep your eyes closed for as long as you can. Remember, no peeking. No touching each other either if there are others near you.

Heartfelt Pledge

Whisper or silently repeat these phrases to yourself after me, "I am healthy and happy." *(Pause.)* "I am talented, just as I am." *(Pause.)* "More and more, I enjoy living." *(Pause.)* "I am protected now." *(Pause.)* "I am loveable, and I am loved, more and more." *(Pause.)* "I can pay attention, stay awake, and practice being alert as I get calmer and calmer."

Physical Relaxation with Imagination

Lift your legs up in the air... Move your legs like you're riding a bike, peddling to one of your favorite places, like to a lake or over to a friend's house... ride harder... and harder... Feel how your legs are working... Now slower... and slower... Oh no, there's an animal in the road. Put the brakes on right now... Good job, you stopped just in time... Go ahead and peddle some more... Now, lower your legs back down for a well-deserved rest... Good job. *(Pause.)*

Bring your knees into your chest, curling up into a ball... Give yourself a nice hug... Stay curled up in a ball... try to make yourself as small as you can... Now, stretch your arms and legs out... reach... make yourself as big as you can... Now, flat as a pancake... Move your arms and hands to your sides.

Pretend you're digging your toes in mud or sand... That's right, scrunch up your toes and stretch them out... Now, swish them around to rinse them off... Let them go back to normal, all clean, all nice and quiet, and feel the difference.

Pretend you are holding colorful balls in both your hands... squeeze them hard... feel how tight your hands and arms are as you squeeze, tighter and tighter... Now, drop the balls... Feel the difference... Once again, squeeze really hard... and drop them and feel the relaxation... Move your fingers and hands out to your sides, just for now. *(Pause.)*

Stretch your arms up into the air... let them fly around like a bird... Do not run into each other, no touching... Be like a bird, soaring and gliding... flying through the warm, bright sunshine... flying through the clouds... And now the bird lands in its nest, nestled and tucked in its nest... Stay real still, so no one knows you're there... still like a statue... Remember, no peeking.

Pretend that someone wants to put a magic carpet under your back... Make some space under there by lifting your back up a few inches... Lower back down and snuggle onto the magic carpet... How big is the magic carpet?... What color is it?... What does it feel like?... Let your body sink into it, all snug.

Wiggle your face all around... and stop, still like a statue... Lift and lower your eyebrows up and down... and stop, still like a statue... Wiggle your nose, like you're a bunny rabbit... and stop, still like a statue... Open your mouth as big as you can and quietly close your mouth a few times ... and stop, still like a statue ... Use your lips like you're blowing bubbles or blowing kisses ... now stop, still like a statue ... Lick your lips if you want ... Close your mouth and keep it closed, like you're going to keep a secret.

Remember to keep your eyes closed. No peeking. Pay attention so you don't miss anything important. Listen carefully. Stay still like a statue.

Breath Awareness

Bring your attention to your nose ... can you feel the air going in and out? ... Let's change it. Listen first, then we'll do it together. Please sniff in through your nose three or so times, like you're smelling a flower and then open your mouth and pretend you're blowing a candle out real fast ... Here you go ... sniff in three times ... and blow out ... sniff in three times ... and blow out ... sniff in three times ... and blow out ... Quit sniffing and blowing and breathe normally for a while. *(Pause.)*

Let's change it. Listen first, then we'll do it together. This time, sniff in three times but breathe out through your nose very slowly. Here you go ... sniff in three times ... and slowly breathe out through your nose ... sniff in three times ... and slowly breathe out your nose ... sniff in three times ... and slowly breathe out your nose ... Quit sniffing and breathe normally for a while. *(Pause.)*

Let's change it again. Listen first, then we'll do it together. This time, instead of sniffing, breathe in through your nose as smoothly as you can and then breathe out through your nose as smoothly as you can. Here you go ... breathe in through your nose, puffing up your belly like it's a balloon ... and slowly let the air all the way out through your nose ... breathe in, filling up your belly like a balloon ... let all the air out as slowly as you can ... breathe in, filling up the balloon ... let all the air out as slowly as you can ... Breathe normally for a while. *(Pause.)*

One last time. Pretend there's a candle in front of you. Take a breath in and blow the candle out ... and make a wish. *(Pause.)*

Superhero Visualization

It's time to use your imagination for a while. Pretend that your favorite superhero has come for a visit. It could be a friend or a protector. It could be from a cartoon or movie. It could be someone you know, or you can make it up. Just so it's a superhero that you can trust and will always watch out for you.

Imagine your superhero now. Let your superhero come to life. What does your superhero look like? ... What is the size of your superhero? ... What is your superhero wearing? ... What kind of voice does your superhero have? ... Imagine your superhero now ...

Your superhero has some messages for you. Here they are. "You are good inside ..." "It's okay to be happy and healthy ..." "You have talents of your own ..." "You are good at learning things ..." "You are loveable, and you are loved."

Gifts and Messages from Superhero

Your superhero has a present for you ... It's a special gift just for you ... Pretend that your superhero hands you a box that's wrapped up in colorful paper and decorated with ribbons and bows. What's the box like? ... Pretend that you are opening it up now ... What's inside? *(Pause.)* Is there a message in it just for you? *(Pause.)* Imagine putting your special gift and message in a safe place, knowing you can use it anytime you want.

Happiness and Joy with Stillness

It's okay to be happy. Imagine feeling happy now with a smile on your face ... If you want, pretend that you're at play, inside or outside ... You can be playing by yourself or with others ... What does it feel like to be happy? ... How does your head and face feel? ... How does happiness feel in your belly? ... How does it feel in your hands and feet? ... Let the feeling of happiness spread all over. *(Pause.)* Remember, there's a place inside of you that is always happy, no matter what's going on ... Let feelings of happiness come alive from within ... Soak happiness up ... Spread it all around.

Heartfelt Pledge and Closing

Either whisper or silently say after me, "I am happy and healthy." *(Pause.)* "I am talented, just as I am." *(Pause.)* "More and more, I enjoy living." *(Pause.)* "I am protected now." *(Pause.)* "I am loveable, and I am loved, more and more." *(Pause.)*

Closing for Waking Up

It's time to wake up. Take a big breath in and sigh it out...take another big breath in and sigh it out... Like a pet waking up, start stretching your arms and legs... Wiggle your arms and legs and body around like a fish... Roll over to your side and curl up like a bug in a rug. *(Pause.)* Use your arms to push yourself up to sit. Open your eyes and smile. The end.

Closing for Going to Sleep

It's time to go to sleep. Imagine there's an invisible blanket of protection covering you up... Make yourself nice and cozy... Good night. It's time to go to sleep. You are loved.

Peace, Peace, Peace. (Om shanti, shanti, shanti.)

Yoga Nidra: Conquer Stress for Teen Empowerment

Contributed by Viviana Collazo

Time: 15–20 minutes is suitable to start. A 30-minute practice is appropriate as attention increases.

Summary: This generation of teens and more mature tweens respond well to the empowering way this Yoga Nidra is offered. It is an excellent technique for teens to reconnect with themselves, to relax, to restore, and to navigate school, work, home life, and extracurricular activities with more confidence, equipping them with positive tools for daily living.

Take enough time for transitioning from getting ready for the practice to doing it. Mudras are used. They are hand gestures used to stimulate vital energy and reestablish a proper direction or flow to the energy of the body. The Pala mudra is offered at the beginning of the session for calming fidgety or anxious feelings and to instill trust. The Kubera mudra is given at the end for integration and to instill a sense of self-confidence and motivation. Mudras can be used anytime, like during the practice and at other times during the day. Both mudras are described in the body of the script. Consider reviewing those instructions beforehand.

Additional Notes: As timesavers, consider eliminating the mudras or the initial breath awareness section. The golden light guided imagery section should be used with care since some teens can be quite sensitive to imagery. It is recommended to omit it if the participant suffers from clinical depression or panic attacks.

Stages	Process / Techniques
Preparation and settling in	Pala mudra hand gesture for calming and trust. Savasana. Focused breath awareness.
Sankalpa	Options given to formulate one's own or use statements given for being calm, happy, loving, brave, or creative.
Physical: Anna-maya kosha	Progressive muscle relaxation with movements
Energetic: Prana-maya kosha	Focused breathing
Mental: Mano-maya kosha	Golden light guided imagery
Intuitive: Vijnana-maya kosha	Intuitive awareness
Bliss: Ananda-maya kosha	Implied experience
True Self: Atman	Implied experience
Sankalpa	Sankalpa with added symbol
Reawakening and closing	Kubera mudra hand gesture for goal setting and confidence

Preparation and Settling In

Begin welcoming yourself into the experience of Yoga Nidra ... As you prepare your space for the practice, make your surroundings quiet and comfortable ... Be sure to turn off all electronic devices and notifications, just for now.

Let's start sitting. We'll get started by using a hand gesture called the Pala mudra. It often helps with calming fidgety feelings and can instill a sense of trust. Please give it a try to see how you like it. Here's how to do it.

- Position your left-hand below the belly button with the palm facing up.
- Position your right-hand palm at the level of the belly button with the palm facing down.
- Keep both palms in a cupped position and a short distance from each other.
- Your hands will be gently touching the abdomen.

- Make sure the shoulders and elbows are relaxed and the spine is in an upright position.
- Practice natural breathing while holding the mudra until you feel settled, perhaps a few minutes.
- Release the mudra.

Transition into lying down on a cushioned mat or bed for Yoga Nidra. It is recommended to use a small pillow under your head. Position your head just high enough so the base of your head rests comfortably on the pillow, making sure the nape of the neck keeps its natural curve and follows a natural alignment with the rest of your spine. This way you can keep the right flow of breath and circulation from the head and through the spine. Another idea is to have a pillow at the back of your thighs to release the lower back and feel more settled in general. Take enough time to make yourself comfortable.

Place your feet about hip width apart, arms to the side, and palms of the hands facing up. If you prefer, you can place your palms facing down.

Yoga Nidra is an experience in deep relaxation while staying fully alert, so try not to fall asleep. Following the directions allows you to gradually go into a state of profound rest while remaining mindful of a process that is effective and at the same time gentle. It's no big deal if you fall asleep, it just works better if you can hover in between being fully awake and sleeping.

You can close your eyes when you feel ready.

Focused Breathing

Begin now to breathe naturally through the nose. With generous attention, follow the flow of breath in and out ... Not trying to change anything in the way you are breathing, rather letting the breath be just as it is for the next few cycles of breathing, in and out.

Now, become aware of the breath around the rim of the nose, and the sensations that accompany the flow of breath on that area for a few breathing cycles ... Be aware of the tingling sensation, the texture, or the temperature of your own breath ... You may sense the cooling, dry, refreshing temperature of the inhalation, followed by the warmer, moist qualities of your exhalation for a few more cycles ... Anytime you get distracted, bring your attention back to the qualities of your breath. *(Pause about 15 seconds.)*

Continue observing a comfortable breath in and out; and with that, allowing yourself to enjoy the moment, here and now, for a few more breathing cycles.

As you continue devoting attention to the way you're breathing, gradually explore other parts of the body in which you notice breath too; maybe the throat... the chest... the belly.

Where do you feel the breath the most inside the body?... Where do you feel expansion and contraction because of the natural movement of the breath? ... Take your time to notice the natural rhythm of breath... and rest your awareness right where it feels most natural to you for a few more breathing cycles.

Sankalpa Setting

As you relax more and more in the awareness of natural breathing... it's now a good time to establish your sankalpa... A sankalpa is a personal resolve, an intention of the highest degree that could bring a positive shift in your life and in the life of others around you. Something you would like to have more and more in your life. A few examples are "I am calm...," "I am happy...," "I enjoy life...," "I love, and I'm loved...," "I am brave...," or "I'm creative."

Take a moment to come up with one of your own, a short, positive statement in the present tense... Simply observe the word or words that come naturally to you as you create your personal resolve. *(Pause.)*

Once you create your sankalpa, repeat it a few times silently, positively and in the present tense. You can add yours to the sentence stem, "I am..."

Dedicate your Nidra meditation practice to that purpose. Let your sankalpa echo through your whole self... and let it go, knowing that results are always according to the highest good of all.

Remember, this experience is one of deep relaxation while your mind remains alert. It is not time to sleep, rather a time to be aware as you are relaxing and breathing comfortably.

Progressive Muscle Relaxation with Movements

Continue settling the body more and more. Be aware of the points of contact your back is making on the surface that supports it... Rely on that support... feeling free at any time to rearrange your position or props if need be.

Let's continue releasing tensions from the body. We can let go of deep buried tensions in the physical body, layer by layer... Please bring your direct attention to the different body regions as they are mentioned.

Starting with attention to your right foot, point and flex your right foot back and forth, activating all the toes, the ankle, lower leg, right knee, higher leg, and hip... and rest... Now slowly lift the whole right leg up a few inches. Hold the engagement for a few seconds, and as you exhale, let it go... Bringing attention now to your left foot. Point and flex your left foot, activating all the toes, the ankle, lower leg, left knee, higher leg, and hip... and rest... Now slowly lift the whole leg up just a few inches. Hold the engagement for a few seconds, and as you exhale, let it go... This time lift both legs at the same time from hip to toes... and let go.

Bringing attention to your right hand, make a fist... Next, uncurl your fingers and stretch them out, activating all fingers, wrist, lower arm, elbow, upper arm, and right shoulder, engaging the whole arm... and rest... Lift it up in the air a few inches. Hold it up for just a few seconds... and as you exhale, let go... Bringing attention to your left hand, make a fist... Next, uncurl your fingers and stretch them out, activating all the fingers, the wrist, lower arm, elbow, upper arm, and left shoulder, engaging the whole arm... rest... Lift it up a few inches, just for a few seconds, and as you exhale, let go... Make a fist with both hands, lifting both arms at the same time now, engaging from the shoulder to fingers... and let go.

Lifting the hips up now by pressing the legs back down, lifting only the hips, and let go... Allow the chest to rise by pressing down the hips and letting the head stay down. Lifting the chest up just a few inches... and let go.

Bringing attention now to your lips, lift them toward your nose, like you are about to kiss your own nose, shrugging eyes, engaging all face muscles, and let go... Stick the tongue out and at the same time breathe out "Ahhh..." Now, moving your jaw side to side, up and down, and let go.

Turning your head side-to-side... try inhaling as you center your head and exhale turning your head to one side... Inhale with moving the head to the center and exhale turning your head slowly to the other side... repeating this a few more times at your own pace.

Returning your head to center, making sure now that you align the jaw with the center of the chest, and relax... How does your neck and shoulders feel now?... Noticing without judgement. *(Pause.)*

Expand your attention to the whole body, exploring how your body feels in general, head to toes... you're fully aware of your body lying down, more at ease... your whole body is more relaxed. *(Pause about 15 seconds.)*

Focused Breathing

If you would like to experience relaxation at a deeper level, begin once again to pay attention to your natural breath. This time noticing the flow of breath around the belly... observing the spontaneous rising and falling movement of the abdomen. Observing the softness of breath along with the gentle movement that it creates in the belly for several breathing cycles. *(Pause.)*

You may silently say, "I'm breathing in" as the belly rises while inhaling, and then you can say, "I'm breathing out" with the outbreath as the belly goes down for several cycles.

After a few times you might prefer a shorter silent statement by only saying, "In" and "Out." Following the natural rhythm of the breath a few more times... belly going up, say "In ...," belly going down, say "Out." Remember to return your focus to your breath each time you catch your attention wandering off. *(Pause about 1 minute.)*

When ready, let go of the words and take your time to enjoy the effects over-all, aware of yourself in a restful moment. *(Pause.)*

Golden Light Guided Imagery

You may continue breathing like this on your own a while longer. If you would like, however, you can choose to relax further. Either imagine, feel, or sense that each breath generates a golden light or a golden liquid or substance that gathers and pools in your abdomen. Be aware of its texture or hue as it presents itself to you... And if you experience a different color than gold, go with what comes naturally to you. Each breath, creating a light, liquid, or substance. *(Pause.)*

This is the essence of vital force. It has the potential of self-balancing, it can help you to further release tightness in the body, soothe away any ache, and dissolve mental stress... It can also replace anything negative that depletes your energy with positive energy, exchanging it into newfound energy so you can replenish and recharge your battery.

Let's continue observing the vital energy filling up and pooling around your abdomen ... One breath at a time ... let it grow in size and radiance ... Notice perhaps a warm sensation around the belly ... The subtle substance gathers until it begins to overflow in a downward direction ... Be aware of your waist and hips ... completely bathed in this light ... then the higher legs, knees, lower legs, ankles, feet, and all toes bathed in vital substance ... feeling its soothing effects smoothing out any muscular tension, and balancing everything on its path. *(Pause.)*

Noticing your lower body, from belly down, completely illuminated within ... You may observe the contrast between the lower body and higher body. Any specific differences? ... Avoiding any judgements, simply recognizing the contrasts, but letting go of any labels, for example: labels of good and bad or comfortable and uncomfortable. Instead practicing neutrality ... just paying neutral attention. *(Pause about a minute.)*

Remember you can rearrange your position or open and close your eyes again at any time, as long as you are being present to your experience in Yoga Nidra.

Now once again, gently return your attention to the energy gathered in your belly ... and let it grow in size and radiance ... As you breathe comfortably, allow the pool in your belly to overflow, but this time moving in an upward direction, traveling to your chest, shoulders, streaming down the arms to the hands and all fingers.

Next, notice the pool in your belly overflowing as the golden substance travels around your waist, to cover your entire back, from lower back to higher back ... Your whole torso, now receiving golden vital essence that not only helps dissolve muscular tensions but also bathes all vital organs, including lungs, heart, and stomach ... Deep within the core of you, enveloped by this soothing golden substance ... watch it illuminate you ... as you receive, you repair and replenish in every way. *(Pause about a minute.)*

You may now give yourself the opportunity to experience the golden essence around your throat and neck ... and your whole face ... the sides of the head, the back of the head, and the top ... your entire head.

Bringing your awareness now to how your brain also receives, until you can sense every part of your skull and brain lighting up by the golden substance... all brain functions, receiving and balancing on all levels.

Give yourself permission now to rest, allowing the effects of the practice so far to take place, fully aware of your experience in the present moment... Enjoy an all-embracing view of your body illuminated, recharging, at ease, resting in the awareness of restoration and peace. *(Pause about 1 minute.)*

This experience in complete tranquility can tune you in on a feeling level too. If you like, pay attention to any emotions or feelings that may arise as a result of this practice... noticing your current feeling state, right at this moment... observing with subtle curiosity, without judging anything of which you become aware. *(Pause.)*

If you wish, you may again use the golden light or substance to help you clear away any challenging emotions by sensing or imagining yourself enveloped and protected by the golden light.

Perhaps picturing a golden blanket wrapping you up and tucking you in... into comfort and loving awareness, allowing and welcoming the healing blanket to surround anywhere: the physical body, the emotional or mental state. This is your practice. You're in charge of your experience at all times. *(Pause about 1 minute.)*

Your consciousness is supported by complete inner stillness... It's happening in the here and now... And in this state of profound relaxation you can access infinite, innate resources, intuitive awareness, and creativity. *(Pause.)*

Sankalpa

Enjoy this quiet space and bring to mind your sankalpa, your personal statement. It carries its own positive and creative vibration. You may repeat your personal statement again a few times...

Let this be felt throughout your whole being... And after a while, let it go... Feel or sense that your entire self becomes the quality you have promoted. *(Pause.)*

You may bring to mind a symbol, image or object that represents that quality, your sankalpa. For example, if you are generating the vibration of happiness, you can use an image of a smile or the memory of a moment in which you lived in pure happiness. Another example is if you are affirming the vibration of courage or confidence, you can bring up an image or symbol that reminds you of being a superhero. Give yourself a moment to come up with your own representation. Let it come from your heart and highest wisdom, trusting the accuracy of your own impression. *(Pause about a minute.)*

You can safely store this quality right inside your heart where it's always readily accessible. *(Pause.)*

Once you return to your daily activities, be aware that you have generated and harnessed positive qualities that will continue serving you as inspiration and guidance throughout the day, and that you are a channel of those qualities as you interact with others, the world, and your everyday life. *(Pause.)*

Reawakening and Closing

You may begin now bringing your attention back to your breath around the nose or your belly, noticing how you feel in general...and inviting yourself to be more alert to your surroundings...in the room...outside the room...letting external sounds arrive and subside as you invite yourself back gradually...letting your body move, wiggling toes and fingers...stretching spontaneously as it comes. *(Pause.)* Letting light filter into your eyes through your eyelids, little by little. *(Pause about 1 minute.)*

When you're ready, roll to one side and stay on your side for a few breaths, enjoying this nurturing position, aware of how you feel for a few more breaths.

Welcome yourself to come back to sitting by pressing your hands down to comfortably come into a full seated position with a tall back. Allow the way you are seated to feel natural and stay mindful of your breath. *(Pause.)*

You're invited to practice the Kubera mudra with your hands. In this case, Kubera mudra helps to energize and seal the energy of your sankalpa and of your practice in general. It instills a sense of self-confidence and motivation after the session. Here's how:

- Rest both hands on your lap.
- With each hand, allow the tip of your thumb, index finger, and the middle finger to unite.
- Bend the pinky finger and ring finger toward the center of the palm.
- Breathe comfortably while holding the mudra.

- Attention can be focused on your sankalpa while doing this. This mudra can also be done throughout the day, especially in connection with sankalpa awareness.

- Hold for a minute or two.

Remember as you return to living your life at home, in school, and during extracurricular activities, you can check in with your breath once in a while. This will help you to stay mindful and to take charge of your day on a positive note. Open your eyes, look around, and notice how you're feeling.

Peace, peace, peace. (Shanti.)

Viviana Collazo, PhD, E-RYT-500, CPYT. Since 1999, Viviana has been dedicated to the holistic field by serving as a Yoga and meditation teacher, energy balancing facilitator, and spiritual counselor in central Florida. As founder and director of the Luminous Holistic Center, she conducts teacher trainings with certification in Yoga, Prenatal Yoga, Reiki, and meditation. She provides seminars in Ayurveda, Vedic philosophy, and dharma studies. Viviana is an ordained minister and earned a doctorate degree through the Alliance of Divine Love International Ministry. Viviana is the mother of two teens and loves spending time with her family. She is a lifelong student and cultivates a playful approach to life by painting and singing.

Welcoming Your Well-Rested Woman: A Daring to Rest Yoga Nidra Meditation

Contributed by Karen Brody

Time: 20–30 minutes

Summary: This Yoga Nidra is designed to help women feel supremely relaxed, safe, grounded, and creative, and that they can take back their power from a rooted place. An invitation to either go to sleep or wake up at the end is given. Uniquely, a touchstone is used. A touchstone is something—real or imaginary—that represents calm, safety, and a sense of grounding throughout Nidra meditation. It could be something from nature, a keepsake like a special ring, or anything that fits into the palm of your hand.

Additional notes: For inclusiveness, substitute "friend," "person," or "sisters and brothers" when feminine references are made when leading a mixed group of women and men.

Chakra energy balancing is included. See appendix 2 for more information about chakras.

Stages	Process / Techniques
Preparation and settling in	Savasana with a touchstone
Sankalpa	Intentions are given for staying awake and being a well-rested woman, or formulating one's own
Physical: Anna-maya kosha	Rotation of consciousness
Energetic: Prana-maya kosha	Breath awareness with guided imagery for well-being and peaceful, joyful rest
Mental: Mano-maya kosha	Chakra energy center visualization

Stages	Process / Techniques
Intuitive: Vijnana-maya kosha	Wisdom council visualization for intuition
Bliss: Ananda-maya kosha	Welcoming waves of joy
True Self: Atman	Pure awareness
Sankalpa	Intention remembrance
Reawakening and closing	Options are given for going to sleep or waking up

Preparation and Settling In

Hello, Rest Sister. It's time to be good to yourself. Daring to Rest begins right now. Throughout Yoga Nidra, you have the choice to follow my voice or not. If there are any instructions you don't wish to follow, you always have the option to return to your touchstone.

If you have an actual touchstone, bring it to your body for a moment... If you don't have an actual touchstone, you're invited to imagine one now... and imagine placing your touchstone, real or imaginary, on or beside your body.

Take a moment now to make sure you're supremely comfortable for Yoga Nidra... Now check in again with your body to see if you could be even more comfortable. *(Pause.)*

Allow the eyes to close... Begin to draw your attention away from any outside noises... and moving awareness now to only your body... and your breath... Take a deep breath in... and exhale with a deep sigh... and again. One more long inhalation... and exhale. *(Pause.)*

Intention

Say to yourself gently, "I will remain awake and aware throughout Yoga Nidra." *(Pause.)* However, if you do fall asleep, know that there is a part of you that is always awake and will hear my voice.

Bring your awareness to the space between your eyebrows. Rest here in stillness. *(Pause.)*

It's time to bring your intention for Yoga Nidra to mind. Your intention is like a seed you wish to plant in your life. You can use the statement, "I am a well-rested woman," or use an intention that resonates deep in your heart. Be sure to state your intention in the present tense, as if it's already happening. Repeat your intention now three times. *(Pause.)*

Rotation of Consciousness

Now take a breath in and, on the exhale, let your body go limp... let go. *(Pause.)*

We will move awareness throughout the body. When you hear a body part named, imagine stress releasing from that area of the body, softening that area of the body even more.

Bring your attention to the right foot, left foot, both feet. Right knee, left knee, both knees. Right hip, left hip, both hips. Right torso, left torso, the whole torso. Right hand, left hand, both hands. Right arm, left arm, both arms. Right shoulder, left shoulder, both shoulders. The neck. Right side of the jaw, left side of the jaw, the whole jaw. Upper lip, lower lip, both lips. The whole mouth. Right cheek, left cheek, both cheeks. Right nostril, left nostril, both nostrils. Right ear, left ear, both ears. Right eye, left eye, both eyes. Right eyebrow, left eyebrow, both eyebrows. Right side of the forehead, left side of the forehead, the whole forehead. Crown of the head. Back of the head. Back of the neck. Upper back, midback, lower back, the whole back. Buttocks. Back of the right leg, back of the left leg, backs of both legs. Heel of the right foot, heel of the left foot, both heels. The whole body... feel the whole body... the whole body is heavy... limp... still. *(Pause.)*

Breath Awareness with Guided Imagery
for Well-Being and Peaceful, Joyful Rest

Bring your attention to the darkness inside your inner eyelids... rest here... If your mind drifts off, allow it. *(Pause.)*

Begin to slowly inhale and allow the exhale to remove tension from your mind and body. *(Pause.)*

Now begin to imagine a golden straw through your body, going from the earth up through your body to your solar plexus, the space just above your navel point, and through the crown of your head to the sky... And imagine breathing in and out through the straw... in... and out. *(Pause.)*

Now, breathing in through the golden straw from earth to the solar plexus and continuing out to the crown of the head to the sky... on the exhale, the breath moves from the sky into the crown of the head, and down to the root of your body, at the base of the spine, and then back to the earth. Inhale through the golden straw, from earth to the solar plexus, and out the crown of the head to the sky... Exhale sky, crown, root, earth... inhale earth, solar plexus, crown, sky... exhale sky, crown, root, earth. Continue breathing like this in your own rhythm...

Now stop... open yourself to whatever arises... Be still and notice sensations in the body... notice your whole body... and see your whole body filling with white healing light... With each breath, white healing light enters the whole body... See yourself lying down, resting, filled with white light. *(Pause.)*

Bring your attention to the space between your eyebrows... let go completely... You are protected. Connected. Grounded... Mother Earth holds you lovingly... Feel yourself completely calm, centered, and present right now. *(Long pause.)*

In this womb of deep rest, welcome in your council of women to be with you. This is a wise council of mentors, guides, living or not, real or imagined, who believe in you. See who comes... And in their loving presence repeat your intention three times. *(Long Pause.)*

Imagine your intention happening and watch them witness your intention. *(Pause.)*

Your council of women may remain, or not, as you slowly deepen your breath into the belly. On the inhale, the breath enters the body through the belly, and on the exhale, the breath exits the body through the belly. Belly breathing. *(Long pause.)*

Experiencing Intuition

On the next inhalation through the belly, follow your breath and allow it to go anywhere in the body. See where it lands and bring your awareness to that area of the body... See if there's an image, word, phrase, or sensation coming from this area—a soul whisper that wants to be known. Be patient... using the exhale to animate whatever you're perceiving, even if it seems like nothing. *(Long pause.)*

Whatever you receive, exhale that soul whisper to your belly. Let it sit at the belly for a moment. Be curious about whatever you received. If you haven't received anything, know that your soul whisper may arrive at the end of Nidra meditation or later on when you're awake or dreaming.

Transitioning into Sleep or Waking Up

If you're going off to sleep, hum or sing yourself to sleep, like a lullaby. *(Pause.)*

If you're waking up, see if there's a song or a hum emerging from your heart...listen...slowly wake yourself up with your voice, or imagine yourself humming, singing softly, the way you'd sing to a baby...your voice waking the body.

The eyes are still closed. Let your body decide what she wants to do next. Maybe that's to move, or not...The mind is quiet. The breath peaceful. The body tranquil. *(Pause.)*

Intention and Closing

Welcome your intention...and notice how it's received in the body. *(Long pause.)*

In her book *Belonging*, Toko-pa Turner says, "There is a wild woman under our skin who wants nothing more than to dance until her feet are sore, sing her beautiful grief into the rafters, and offer the bottomless cup of her creativity as a way of life. And if you are able to sing from the very wound that you've worked so hard to hide, not only will it give meaning to your own story, but it becomes a corroborative voice for others with a similar wounding."[22] *(Pause.)*

If you're waking up, slowly open your eyes. As you come back, begin to imagine taking the fruits of deep rest back into your life.

Wake like a well-rested woman, intentionally, consciously, with deep awareness that you are enough. You are worthy. You are whole and complete no matter what. No one—no force—can take your power away from you.

This completes Daring to Rest. It's time to go to sleep or to stretch...roll to your side...and begin the journey back to waking.

Be good to yourself, Rest Sister.

Karen Brody is a mother and the founder of Daring to Rest, whose mission is to create a world of well-rested people. Using

---

22. Toko-pa Turner, *Belonging: Remembering Ourselves Home* (Salt Spring Island, British Columbia: Her Own Room Press, 2017), 94.

her Yoga Nidra framework, the Daring to Rest method is particularly focused on training women in Yoga Nidra meditation and supporting women to personally use Yoga Nidra to reclaim their power. Visit Karen's website at daringtorest.com for more.

Resources

Brody, Karen. *Daring to Rest: Reclaim Your Power with Yoga Nidra Rest Meditation, a 40-Day Program for Women.* Boulder, Colorado: Sounds True, 2017.

Yoga Nidra for Men's Health

Julie Lusk

Time: 20–30 minutes

Summary: This Yoga Nidra experience is geared for furthering overall health for men and women by offloading stress to regulate the nervous system using muscular tension and release. Options are given for either progressive muscle relaxation (PMR) or for lifting and dropping portions of the body to accommodate preferences and contraindications as outlined on page 256 in appendix 4. Breath control, mental focus, and more are included. It can be used to refuel one's energy and resilience, increase heart health, improve sleep quality, and increase concentration. Options are given for customizing the experience to meet one's own needs. The terminology used is direct and to-the-point.

Stages	Process / Techniques
Preparation and settling in	Savasana
Sankalpa	Heartfelt pledge for courage, insight, or a self-selected quality to enhance well-being
Physical: Anna-maya kosha	Options for progressive muscle relaxation or lifting and dropping portions of the body
Energetic: Prana-maya kosha	Breath awareness and measured breathing to reset the nervous system
Mental: Mano-maya kosha	Mindfulness training and guided imagination using a solvent to dissolve stressful thoughts and feelings

Stages	Process / Techniques
Intuitive: Vijnana-maya kosha	Advisory team visualization for guidance and experiencing instinctual, intuitive understanding
Bliss: Ananda-maya kosha	Guided imagination, unconditional joy, and true nature awareness
True Self: Atman	Pure awareness (implied)
Sankalpa	Heartfelt pledge
Reawakening and closing	

Preparation and Settling In

This is a time to investigate, identify, and unload tension and pressure. Doing so will help unleash pent up energy, charge up your body, and strengthen your mind and spirit.

Kick back for a while. Lie down on your back or sit in a comfortable chair. Choose a place that feels stable and supportive. Cover up to maintain body warmth. Depending on your position and preference, you can use a thin pillow under your head to protect the curve at the back of the neck. Too much of an angle between your head and neck might hinder blood flow so only tuck your chin slightly. Perhaps put a large, sturdy pillow or rolled up blanket beneath your thighs for leg and back support. Align the center of your chin with the center of your chest. Uncross your arms and legs. Check it all out…Now, feel free to move around until you're most comfortable…Follow along with as much or as little attention as you want, giving your innermost needs some room for expression. Either close your eyes or let them be partially open…You're in charge of this experience.

Heartfelt Pledge

You're invited to have an intention (sankalpa). This powerful tool enriches your Yoga Nidra experience and transfers its benefits into daily life. It's a positive trait to build your skills at home or work, in sports, or in the arts. It's a foundation for living a meaningful life. Examples are, "I have courage," or "I have insight."

There's no need to rush into this. Perhaps the one that's right for you isn't ready to show itself yet. If so, be open to having it come when the time is right. When it does, you will know it and feel that it's genuine and true for you. If yours isn't apparent, rest assured that a deep part of your real self always has your best interest at heart and is already working on your behalf.

Either use the intention you already have or let something occur to you… Keep it straightforward, positive, and to the point. Say it in the present tense as if it's already happening… It may have a symbol or emblem to represent it… Say it silently to yourself a few times. *(Pause.)* Take a big breath in… and let it go.

Progressive Muscle Relaxation

Let's resolve some physical tension first by systematically tensing and releasing muscle groups. If you prefer or need to, lift and drop instead of tensing as we go along.

Bring your attention to your entire right leg. Begin tensing or lifting it as strongly as you want… feeling all that effort… Now release it… and let the muscles become effortless, just for now… Next, bring your attention to your entire left leg. Begin tensing or lifting it as strongly as you want… feeling all that effort… Now release it… and let the muscles become effortless, just for now… Take a big breath in and sigh it out.

This time target your attention on both of your shoulders, arms, and hands. Lifting them up or making strong fists, curling your fingers into a tight ball… compress the muscles in your arms and shoulders and hold it… spread your fingers out… and release… dissolving all that tension, like ice melts from the heat of the sun… Take a big breath in and sigh it out. *(Pause.)*

Bring your attention to your torso… Begin by lifting your back up from what it's on to tense from your glutes to your upper back. Hold it… release it all… notice if your back automatically presses firmly onto the surface that's supporting you from behind… Feel free to let that sink in… Now, tense your stomach and chest or imagine doing so, noticing all that effort, all that pressure… hold on… and let go, perhaps feeling the relief of discharging all that pressure and tension… welcoming in a sense of ease and effortlessness, just for now. Take a big breath in and sigh it out. *(Pause.)* Simply breathing naturally and effortlessly for now. *(Pause.)*

Now it's time to tense and release your face and head, or imagine it. First, press your tongue against the back of your teeth or the roof of your mouth ... release ... Press your lips together ... release ... Lift the corners of your lips up ... release ... Press the corners of your lips down ... release ... Let the corners of your lips become neutral, more and more ... moisten your lips if you want, and let your entire mouth rest. There's no need to speak, answer to anyone, or say anything, out loud or silently. It's okay to be quiet ... If distractions happen, let them move on out, shoveling them all away. *(Pause.)*

With your eyes closed, lift and lower your eyebrows ... and let them rest, allowing the area around your eyes to smooth out, like when lake water smooths completely out and becomes reflective ... still and reflective.

And a clear liquid stream washes through you, rinsing away any remnants of tension, relieving pressure, and cleaning out what's no longer needed ... naturally repairing and rebuilding from the inside out ... It's refreshing.

And scanning your body from the top, down through the middle, and all the way out to your fingers and toes, noticing what's happening, whatever it is. *(Pause.)*

Measured Breathing

Please target your attention on your breath. This will steady your energy by smoothing out static. When you're ready, begin noticing how your breath is simply and naturally coming and going in and out ... there's no need to change or fix it ... focusing attention on your breath as it comes and goes ... exercising your concentration skills as you continue following your breath during the pause. *(Pause.)*

Let's drill down even more by only paying attention to inhaling ... noticing each breath as it goes in ... again and again ... When you're ready, begin measuring the inhalation by counting the duration of each inhalation (it's okay if it changes), simply counting the duration of every inhalation during the quiet pause. *(Pause about 30 seconds.)*

And now, what's the average number for the time it takes to inhale? ... From here, continue breathing in for that amount of time and start to lengthen your exhalation. So, if you're breathing in for four or five, begin breathing out for five to ten, making sure that the inhalation and exhalation match or that the exhalation is longer. Counting while breathing in and breathing out for that number or more ... there's no need to hurry ... Start with a fresh breath each time you get distracted, targeting attention onto breathing and counting. Remember to return attention to the breath each time it wanders during the pause. *(Pause about 1-2 minutes.)*

Mindfulness Training with Guided Imagination

If you like, you may want to shed another layer by turning attention to your thoughts and mood. Allowing your thoughts and beliefs, your moods, feelings, or emotions to come and go ... giving them some room ... knowing there's nothing you have to do about it ... simply letting them appear, be, and eventually disappear. *(Pause.)*

Perhaps you'd like to come to a place that's clear of thoughts and feelings. If so, imagine there's a solvent, liquid, or gas that can easily and safely dissolve whatever's not needed, dissolving distractions. It's something that clears and cleans out the gunk ... outdated thoughts and feelings evaporate ... it vaporizes the to-do list ... it releases the pressure valve ... So, when distractions or annoyances occur, this solvent takes care of it ... clearing out and letting anything that gets in the way disappear into the solvent during this silence. *(Pause about 1–2 minutes.)*

Checking in with yourself, from a place that's curious and impartial ... checking in with your body ... your hands ... your gut ... your chest ... head and face ... Checking in with your thoughts and feelings ... Checking in. *(Pause.)*

Now letting all this go for a little while. Clearing the space for being in the moment, being with whatever's happening, watching from a place that's from your core, your bona fide inner core. *(Pause about 1–2 minutes.)*

Experiencing Instinctual, Intuitive Understanding

Somehow, there's a team of advisors here for you. It could be anything at all: a person, an animal, a force of nature, or something mystical. Old or new, real or imaginary. They're your fans. It's a team who has your best interest at heart, willing and able to provide some coaching and guidance. *(Pause.)*

If you like, you may allow a message to appear on its own or, perhaps, ask a question ... allowing something to surface ... Perhaps there's something that you could do or stop doing. *(Pause.)* Perhaps there's something you could say or not say. *(Pause.)* Using this time to be with your team of advisors. *(Pause about 1–2 minutes.)*

This team is always available, always ready and willing to assist you with whatever is needed, as constant as the North Star. *(Pause.)*

Unconditional Joy and True Nature Awareness

Now the solvent starts dissolving whatever roles and responsibilities you have, just for now…It frees up who you really are at your core, your authentic Self… it's the durable aspect that gets to the meat of who you really are; spacious, open, and free.

Take this time of quiet for your true Self. *(Pause about 1–2 minutes.)*

Heartfelt Pledge

It's time to recall your intention, your own pledge (sankalpa), if you have one. Say it briefly and sincerely. *(Pause.)* Let yourself imagine what it looks and feels like…Take a big breath in…and sigh it out. *(Pause.)*

Reawakening and Closing

It's time to bring your awareness back to this time and place, bringing back with you the helpfulness of the practice to benefit yourself and others…Becoming aware of the room…sensing the atmosphere…listening to the sounds…being aware of your Presence…awakening…here and now…

Whenever you're ready, start to stretch in ways that feel natural…Gradually roll to your side and rest…Gradually, use your arms for support to sit yourself upright…As your eyes open, notice whatever you're experiencing.

Peace, peace, peace. (Om shanti, shanti, shanti.)

A Beginning iRest Yoga Nidra Script for Active Duty Service Members, Veterans, Families, Health Care Providers, and Support Staff

Contributed by Robin Carnes

Time: 35–45 minutes

Summary: This script focuses on reducing stress-related symptoms like pain, insomnia, anxiety, and anger issues using evidence-based practices to regulate the autonomic nervous system by activating the parasympathetic nervous system (relaxation response). This is usually helpful for anyone experiencing the stress of being a human being. It is appropriate for those with post-traumatic stress, military sexual trauma, or secondary traumatic stress.

Several breathing techniques are offered. Use all of them or choose fewer depending on one's needs and the amount of time available.

If used in a group, you may ask if anyone wants to share something about their experience afterward, with the reminder there is no way to have done it wrong. It is important to be available later to answer questions or for those who would like to share more privately.

Additional Notes: Important instructions are given for leading individuals and groups of active duty service members and veterans in appendix 4. It is strongly advised that a meditation teacher, Yoga instructor, or therapist undertake specialized training in military-informed wording and trauma-informed approaches before working with members of our military community. Without proper training, unintentional harm may occur when working with people who have trauma or traumatic brain injury (TBI) in their backgrounds. See the resource list at the end of this script for training opportunities.

Stages	Process / Techniques
Preparation and settling in	Relaxation pose (lying down or sitting in a chair) and welcoming messengers
Sankalpa	Intentions for this practice Heartfelt desire Inner resource
Physical: Anna-maya kosha	Welcoming body sensations with witnessing and rotation of consciousness
Energetic: Prana-maya kosha	Breath sensing and breath counting
Mental: Mano-maya kosha	Welcoming and witnessing emotions, feelings, thoughts, and beliefs
Intuitive: Vijnana-maya kosha	Welcoming and witnessing; cognitions
Bliss: Ananda-maya kosha	Joy and equanimity
Being whole: Sahaj	Welcoming well-being, whatever is present
True Self: Atman	Everything just as it is
Sankalpa	Heartfelt desire and intentions
Reawakening and closing	Taking the practice into the world

Preparation and Settling In

The intent of this meditation is *not* to "try to relax." Rather, the intent is to simply observe and welcome sensations in the body and breath with a curious and friendly attitude. When we "try to relax," the goal of controlling our experience can actually create more tension. So, this exercise is an experiment in not trying to change anything, but rather witnessing and feeling what is happening moment-to-moment in the body with as much curiosity and friendliness toward yourself as possible.

Let's gather some "before" data first. Right now, if you were to rate your anxiety level on a scale of 0 to 10, with 0 being low and 10 being high, what would it be? ... Right now, if you were to rate your level of physical discomfort or pain, on a scale of 0 to 10, what would it be? ... We'll check again on these scales when we complete the practice to see how it affected you.

Remember, we are not trying to relax or change anything. We are not looking for a particular outcome, just gathering data in an experiment. If something I ask you during this meditation isn't noticeable to you or just doesn't make sense, just ignore it and wait for the next instruction. Remember that at any time you feel like stopping this for any reason, you can. You are in charge.

I will be inviting you to notice different things, primarily feelings in the body. Whenever your attention wanders off from where I'm pointing you, don't worry. Simply and gently reorient back to the things I'm suggesting. If your body falls asleep, that's okay. If it doesn't, that's okay too. If you hear every word, fine. If you hear almost nothing, that's fine too. You really can't do this wrong. When practicing iRest Yoga Nidra, less strain equals more gain.

Go ahead and get comfortable in your chair or on the floor. Allow yourself to be supported by the surface beneath you. I invite you to close your eyes, or you may keep them open if that is more comfortable. My eyes will stay open the entire time, and I will remain aware of the room we are in. I'll have a view of the door at all times.

Sankalpa

Intentions for This Practice

Let's start by just breathing deeply and turning your awareness inward... Feel the sensation of your breath as it passes in and out through your nose. *(Pause.)*

Checking in with yourself about why you are doing this practice... Is it curiosity? Wanting to feel better? Some rest? What is your honest reason or intention for practicing today? Notice that intention, whatever it is. *(Pause.)*

Sankalpa for Your Heartfelt Desire

And now paying attention to your heart with an easy focus... inviting in clarity about what you care about most... What is your deepest heartfelt longing or desire?... What is more important to you than all else?... What quality or value is most important?... What is your heartfelt mission in this life?... Letting this come to you... feeling yourself as a living expression, right now, of this that you are most devoted to... feeling it in your body now. *(Pause 20 seconds.)*

Sankalpa for Your Inner Resource

And inviting in your inner resource … Your inner resource is a scene or a memory in which you felt comfortable and at ease being just as you are … could be a moment in childhood, or time spent with a friend, or pet, or a family member you love or loved, and who loved you … Could be a place in nature you love to be … or it could be an experience, doesn't need to be anything peak or profound. Just a moment when you felt okay or a sense of well-being. Like in that moment, you were in harmony with life.

It's also normal if nothing came to you, no idea of an inner resource today. That happens to many folks for the first time or two. Just be open, don't worry about it, and something will show up as something good to relive. And you may also have more than one inner resource. It may change from time to time.

Now relive this moment, if one has come to you, and experience its visual aspects: the light, colors, shapes … let this all come to you, what it looks like in this scene … then the sounds that are a part of it, let them come to you as if they are happening right now … and the tastes and smells that are a part of it, experiencing them now … and the way this moment, living this experience, feels in your body … in your legs and feet … in your belly … in your chest … around your heart … in your arms and hands … feeling the experience of this comfort and ease, this experience of nothing to prove, nothing else needed to be just right. *(Pause.)*

You can come back to this inner resource any time during the practice. You can ignore my words and come back to it anytime. I'll be inviting it back in several times as well. It's always there for you, this inner resource.

Welcoming Body Sensations with Witnessing

Now we will take a journey through your physical body. I'll name one part of the body at a time. Just let your attention softly focus there and feel into it. If you want, you can wiggle the different parts of the body as they are called out. This may help you sense that part more easily and help you remain focused throughout the exercise. Do what feels right in your body for this exercise … not trying to change what you notice, just feel what is happening there already. No way to do it wrong.

Feel the soles of the feet … left … and then right … feeling both feet … observing the sensation of your feet resting on the surface beneath you.

Now sense the lower legs...the knees...the thighs, left and right...Feel just the left leg, foot, and toes...Now, just the right leg, foot, and toes...Now both legs, feet, and toes...

Now feel the torso...Notice sensation in your belly...Notice sensation in your back...Feel your lower back...mid-back...and upper back.

Bring your attention to the sensation in your left thumb...Feel the sensation in the rest of your fingers on your left hand...notice the sensation in your left palm...now the whole left hand...Bring your attention to the sensation in your right thumb...Feel the sensation in the rest of your fingers on your right hand...notice the sensation in your right palm...feel the whole right hand...Turn your awareness to both hands, sensing both hands at the same time...Now both arms, sensing left and right at the same time...Now your arms, hands, and fingers simultaneously. *(Pause.)*

Now noticing your head...Feel any sensations in the mouth...feel the teeth...the gums...the left inner cheek...the right inner cheek...in and around the tongue...sensations in the entire mouth...Sensation in the left ear...right ear...inner and outer ears...Sensations in and around the left eye...the right eye...all the sensations in and around both eyes...Sensing the nostrils, left and right...the bridge of the nose and the entire nose...Sensing the skin on your face...Can you feel any movement of air across your face?...Feeling the sensations of the entire head. *(Pause.)*

And accessing the inner resource once again...inviting that "in your body" feeling of security and comfort and ease. *(Pause.)*

And now dropping back into awareness and sensing the whole body...feel the whole body as alive sensations, the whole body...observing any places in your body that are particularly noticeable. Feeling all the changing sensations in the body...noticing how all the sensations are always moving and changing.

And now orienting attention to the part of you that has been noticing all this...feeling into aware Presence itself that's always in the background...letting that noticing presence come gently into the foreground and sensing into it...What does it feel like being aware? *(Pause.)*

Breath Sensing

Now turning attention to your breath by noticing that your body is breathing...If you can, breathe through your nose, if not, your mouth is fine too.

Feel the breath coming in and leaving the body, not thinking about it, just simply notice that your body is already breathing and notice how that feels right now. *(Pause.)*

Noticing the feeling of the inside of your nostrils or mouth as the breath goes in and out...As the breath goes in and out, it creates sensation in the inside of the nostrils or mouth. Without straining, see if you can feel that sensation, whatever it is. *(Pause.)*

Deepening Breath Sensing

Now focusing especially on the outbreath, the exhale...How does that feel inside the nostrils or mouth?...Now focusing especially on the inbreath, the inhale...How does that feel inside the nostrils or mouth?

Do you notice any difference in the sensation of the inhale and the exhale?...Not trying to make something happen, just noticing what is already happening right this moment. *(Pause.)*

Now noticing the feeling of the breath as it passes through the back of the throat...How does that feel right now?...Now noticing the movement of the chest as you breathe...even if it's subtle, can you sense some movement in the chest or side ribs? No need to find words, just noticing the sensations as they come and go. Curious about the rhythm of the breath...Is it even and predictable?...Uneven?...Slow?...Fast?

Now noticing the length of the inhale compared to the length of the exhale ...Is the inhale longer, the same length, or shorter than the exhale?...However it is happening is just fine. *(Pause.)*

Now noticing the movement of the abdomen as you breathe...If you can't feel any movement of the abdomen, that is normal, but if you do, what does it feel like in this moment? *(Pause.)*

Breath Counting with Witnessing

Now counting the breaths. Counting exhales only. Starting at six and counting back to zero. At zero, go back to six, counting again back to zero. One count for each exhalation. Here's how: on the next exhalation, count six, inhale naturally, then exhale, count five, and so on. If there's a mistake, or forgetting, just go back to six and keep counting exhales at the abdomen...Attention gently at the abdomen as the body inhales and exhales and there is counting backward. *(Leave about two to three minutes of counting breaths with reminders of "just counting and breathing" every 20–30 seconds.)*

And letting the counting go ... continuing to feel the breath coming and going. And bringing in the feeling of the inner resource ... accessing the feeling in the body of comfort and ease ... throughout the body. *(Pause.)*

And noticing how all the sensations of breath keep changing on their own ... coming and going ... easy and slow sensations coming and going.

And now orienting attention to the part of you that has been noticing all this ... feeling into aware Presence itself, always in the background ... letting that noticing Presence come gently into the foreground and sensing into it. What does it feel like being aware?

Welcoming and Witnessing Emotions, Feelings, Thoughts, and Beliefs

And noticing any sensations of coolness in the body. Scanning the body and noticing the places that already feel a bit cool relative to the rest of the body ... And noticing places in the body that feel warmer ... Tuning in to warm sensations with a friendly curiosity ... and sensing the coolness ... and the warmth ... And now opening up into sensing the warmth and coolness simultaneously. Feeling both at the same time. The mind cannot do this. Dropping back into the part of you feeling both, feeling both ... and noticing how this feels, noticing anything that has changed or shifted.

And noticing if any emotions, thoughts, or beliefs are present right now ... pleasant or unpleasant, it doesn't matter ... Sensing into whether an emotion, thought, or belief, or even an image is arising. Noticing that ... nothing to change. Nothing to do. Witnessing whatever is happening without necessarily engaging. What would it feel like to allow everything to be as it is?

And if there is something arising, where do you notice its sensation in the body? ... Not having to engage with it, just sensing into where it shows up in the body ... Just noticing its presence or absence and the feeling in the body. *(Pause.)*

And accessing the inner resource at any time it feels right ... feeling it in the body. Inviting in any existing quality of well-being or feeling okay or comfort in this moment. No need to create or force anything ... just seeing if this good feeling might be already present in this moment and noticing how it feels in the body. *(Pause 1 minute.)*

Welcoming Underlying Well-Being or Whatever is Present

And welcoming whatever is arising. No way to feel it wrongly or do it wrongly. Just allowing everything to unfold on its own.

And now noticing the feeling of being aware once again... dropping back into the experience of being awareness itself... letting thinking and analyzing go and just feeling back into that part of you that is always awake and aware and welcoming life as it happens... Feeling the experience in this moment of being aware itself... just aware presence... nothing to do or make happen... just the feeling of being. *(Pause.)*

Setting your body sensations free to be as they are... setting your mind and thoughts to be as they are... your emotions free to come and go... and resting in this open, spacious sense of being that never changes. *(Pause 30–60 seconds.)*

And accessing your inner resource whenever and if ever that feels right. *(Pause.)*

Heartfelt Desire, Intentions, and Closing

And noticing this journey you've been on through the feeling of being... the experience of noticing well-being, exploring thoughts, emotions, images, and beliefs as things that come and go in your awareness... breathing... and the physicality of the body... the firm, dense heaviness of the body on the floor or in the chair... Noting your inner resource and your heartfelt desire and the intention you had for this practice.

And imagining yourself going back into your day or evening taking with you this sense of Being and well-being... always there... responding to life in the moment... in harmony with yourself and life... how that feels... perhaps an action you want to take or something that needs to be said or not said... just noticing.

And feeling the body again, perhaps a heavy sensation... starting to transition... noticing the breath and starting to breathe more deeply in the next few minutes... Perhaps wiggling fingers and toes... and taking your time to transition for the next couple of minutes. Stretching in ways that feel natural. *(Pause 2–3 minutes or longer.)*

And if you're lying down, roll over to your side when you're ready…and eventually using your arms for support to come up to sitting. *(Pause 2–3 minutes for sitting.)*

Right now, if you were to rate your anxiety level on a scale of 0 to 10, what would it be?…Right now, if you were to rate your level of physical discomfort or pain on a scale of 0 to 10, what would it be?

Slowly opening your eyes when you're ready. Thank you for your willingness and your openness to participate.

Robin Carnes is a leader in bringing evidence-based Yoga and meditation practice into mainstream settings such as the Department of Defense, VA, and universities. From 2006–2012, Robin was a Yoga and meditation instructor for a DOD acute PTSD program at Walter Reed Medical Center. She cofounded Warriors at Ease, which has trained over one-thousand Yoga teachers to work safely and effectively in military communities. Featured in the *Washington Post, Woman's Day Magazine, Huffington Post, and Army Magazine,* as well as the award-winning documentary, *Escape Fire: The Fight to Rescue American Healthcare.* Robin was honored by the Smithsonian Institution for her pioneering work. Visit RobinCarnes.com and WarriorsAtEase.org for more.

Resources

For training to work with military members, veterans and their families: http://warriorsatease.org

For teacher training in iRest: http://irest.org

For research on iRest: https://www.irest.org/irest-research

For research on meditation for military members, go to http://warriorsatease.org/resources/research/

Carnes, Robin and Terry B. Northcut. "Beginning with the Clients: Mindfully Reconciling Opposites with Survivors of Trauma/Complex Traumatic Stress Disorders." In *Cultivating Mindfulness in Clinical Social Work*, edited by Terry B. Northcut, 103–128. Cham, Switzerland: Springer International Publishing, 2017.

FIVE

Health and Well-Being

THIS CHAPTER IS DEDICATED to Yoga Nidra meditations appropriate for easing anxiety, depression, pain, insomnia, as well as for other health conditions. In addition, they are helpful in generating and maintaining good health in general.

I AM Yoga Nidra for Health and Healing–Kamini Desai

A series of body, breath, and awareness techniques are used to remove mental and emotional disturbance and awaken self-healing. In a profound state of restful awareness, the seeds of inner conflict and disease can be resolved at their root, facilitating healing shifts in the body, and rebalancing mind and emotions.

Yoga Nidra for Restoring and Enhancing Health and Well-Being–Julie Lusk

Autogenic training, healing breath, guided imagination for enhancing immunity and cell regeneration, and health-enhancing intuitive guidance come together to generate deep calmness. Guided imagination for remembering wellness is incorporated.

Yoga Nidra and Self-Healing, California College of Ayurveda–Marc Halpern

Rotation of consciousness, healing sankalpas, and visualization are used for healing.

Healing Chakra Chorus–Jennifer Reis

Body sensing using the rotation of consciousness, breath, color, and nature images are used to balance the chakras (energy centers). An imagined "healing flower" is mentally placed throughout the body (nyasa) and then complemented with chanting aum.

Bihar Yoga Nidra: Intermediate Chakra Visualization–Swami Shankardev Saraswati

This intermediate practice is a dharana (concentration) practice and part of a series of Yoga Nidra techniques that gradually unfold an authentic experience of the chakras and the psychic body. It starts the process of purifying the subtle body and awakening the chakras into consciousness. Rotation of consciousness and breathing to awaken chakras are included.

Sleep Well with Yoga Nidra–Julie Lusk

Sensory awareness, rotation of consciousness, and guided imagination are used. Brushing techniques are done to clear physical, mental, and emotional issues for a good night's sleep.

Calm Frazzled Nerves, Anxiety, and Ease Exhaustion with LifeForce Yoga Nidra–Rose Kress

An imaginary inner sanctuary, a sensory rotation of consciousness, side-to-side breathing, and awareness of opposites are used. Heartfelt awareness nurtures unconditional love and acceptance.

Lifting Depression and Energy with LifeForce Yoga Nidra–Amy Weintraub

Rotation of consciousness coupled with specialized breathing and the awareness of opposites are used to help regulate mood. The ability to accept whatever mood is visiting, and knowing it will change, increases so an improved sense of well-being and joy can be experienced.

iRest Yoga Nidra Meditation for
Chronic Pain Relief–Stephanie Lopez

Nonjudgmental welcoming, a three-part sankalpa, rotation of consciousness with breath, sensing opposites, and using color are implemented to peel away labels to meet pain as pure sensation with awareness. Autonomic nervous system regulation, building self-compassion, and enhancing a sense of meaning and purpose are cultivated and useful for living with pain.

I AM Yoga Nidra for Health and Healing

Contributed by Kamini Desai

Time: Variable. This script is about 35 minutes, depending on the number of affirmations used.

Summary: The energy based Integrative Amrit Method of Yoga Nidra (I AM Yoga Nidra) is known for releasing the healing potential of the body and creating the most profound states of Yoga Nidra quickly. Healing shifts in the body, inner harmony, and rebalancing the mind and emotions are facilitated. The quieter the mind becomes, the more energy is freed to carry out its rejuvenating and restorative functions.

Yogic breath and tension reduction are highlighted to stimulate the relaxation response and initiate healing. The awareness of opposites technique is used, which, according to yogis, helps in gaining control over the involuntary nervous system, which plays an important role in regulating major bodily functions. Inflammation and cortisol decrease, serotonin increases, and the immune and endocrine systems improve. You will become progressively more stress and anxiety resistant as these positive biological effects accumulate.

This profound state of restful awareness accelerates healing in any area of the body by resolving sources of inner conflict and disease at their root. Intentions are used to plant seeds of change in a state of whole brain listening. Eight weeks of daily practice improves brain function for depression and anxiety. After eleven hours of daily practice, you will have boosted functioning in the part of the brain that increases emotional intelligence and the ability to manage fear.[23] Pain, insomnia, low energy, exhaustion, or burnout are minimized.

---

23. Sara W. Lazar et al., "Meditation Experience Is Associated with Increased Cortical Thickness," 1893–1897.

Additional Notes: A list of affirmations is offered. Use up to three affirmations or repeat one affirmation three times. Give time to let each affirmation be absorbed.

Stages	Process / Techniques
Preparation and settling in	Savasana and internalization
Sankalpa	Healing affirmations
Physical: Anna-maya kosha	Deliberate tension and relaxation with option of lifting and dropping portions of the body
Energetic: Prana-maya kosha	Bumblebee breath and complete yogic breath
Mental: Mano-maya kosha	Awareness of opposites; heavy and light
Intuitive: Vijnana-maya kosha	Integration, intention, affirmations, and imagery for guidance
Bliss: Ananda-maya kosha	Witnessing
True Self: Atman	Awareness of higher Self
Sankalpa	Intentions and affirmations
Reawakening and closing	Externalizing

Internalize

Close your eyes and quiet your mind... be still... Let go of all thoughts, worry, and tension... give yourself fully to a higher power... Relax, trust, and let go... Breathe in fully and exhale with a deep sigh... and again, breathe in fully and exhale with a deep sigh... and let go even more... Feel a deep sense of contentment and peace in your heart. *(Pause.)*

Deliberate Tension and Relaxation

We will move our attention into the body to release trapped energy and move deeper into total relaxation. Those with cardiac disease, hypertension, or glaucoma should use caution. If you cannot have undue pressure in the head for any reason, it is important that you breathe normally and only lightly tense the body. If you prefer, you may lift the named area slightly followed by dropping it.

As you inhale, make fists, and deliberately induce stiffness and tension throughout your shoulders, arms, and fists ... tighten ... tighten ... even more ... Now let go completely ... relax.

On your next exhalation, relax even more ... let go ... observe and feel the flood of energy in your arms. *(Pause.)*

This time, as you inhale, deliberately induce stiffness and tension in the hips, legs, and feet. Tighten ... tighten ... hold ... hold. Let go. Let go completely. Relax ... observe the flood of energy in your legs. *(Pause.)*

This time tighten and tense the entire body as you inhale ... hands, arms, shoulders, feet, legs, face ... tighten ... tighten ... Now let go completely ... relax.

On your next exhalation let go even more ... Observe and feel the energy extending to all the muscles, nerves, and cells of your entire body ... Release any holding anywhere. *(Pause.)*

Bumblebee Breath

This next phase is to enter into deeper and subtler levels of relaxation through the bumblebee sound and breath. In a moment, we will take a deep breath in and, with closed lips, we will begin to hum the sound of the bumblebee. Place the tongue where the roof of the mouth touches the upper teeth. Change the pitch of the buzzing sound to maximize the vibratory sensation felt in your skull. Use your thumbs to gently close your ears, just tight enough so that you can still hear. Rest the remaining fingers on either side of the forehead.

Now, take a breath in and hum ... Mmmmmmmm. *(Allow up to 7 breaths.)* Now stop ... bring your arms by your sides ... and be still.

Bring your total undivided attention to your whole body ... feel the stimulating impact of the vibrations extending throughout your whole body ... observe your energy field, expanding and growing ... extending everywhere and filling every nerve and cell of your body. *(Pause.)*

Now bring your attention to the eyebrow center ... and empty your mind into the flood of energy ... Drop into complete silence and deep stillness. *(Pause.)*

Universal Instructions

As this next phase of Yoga Nidra is entered, remain as motionless as possible. If you need to move or make an adjustment, do so mindfully, returning to stillness as soon as you are able. Resolve to remain awake, staying in touch with the sound of my voice. Allow your entire body to respond directly and non-mentally to my words. Allow any disturbances, external or internal, to draw you more deeply within.

Now shift from thinking and doing to feeling and being ... Do absolutely nothing from now on ... Drop into the deepest state of tranquility, stillness, and peace in the third eye center between the eyebrows. *(Pause.)*

Now your consciousness is in direct communion with your energy body. *(Pause.)*

Complete Yogic Breath

Now follow my guidance as we begin the relaxation breath ... Breathing in deeply, fill your lungs from the bottom to the top as if you are filling a water bottle. As you breathe out, empty your lungs from the top to the bottom. Let your breath be slow and steady ... observe the movement of your abdomen and chest. *(Pause.)*

Stay connected to the wonderful feeling of the release of tension and the deep feeling of relaxation ... Let this feeling extend to every part of your body ... Let this entire process of breathing be the vehicle for deepening your relaxation. *(Pause.)*

Now redirect your full attention to your breath ... bring your undivided attention to the movement of your abdomen and chest as you breathe in and out ... Create no struggle around breathing; use the breath to release any tensions ... Let the flow of your breath be steady and uniform as much as possible. *(Pause.)*

With each breath out, release any tension held in your body ... Anticipations in your mind let go ... With each breath in, fill every nerve and cell with pulsating, healing energy. *(Pause.)*

Now breathe normally and be still. *(Pause.)*

Bring your total attention to the energy field felt in the form of sensations in your body ... let all the tension simply melt, drain away, and dissolve in the expanding energy field.

Bring your attention to your eyebrow center ... empty your body and mind and enter deeper levels of stillness and silence. *(Pause.)*

Do absolutely nothing from now on ... Settle into the silent Source of your being. *(Pause.)*

Awareness of Heavy and Light Sensations

As each body part is named, bring your total attention to it accompanied by a feeling of heaviness, sinking like a stone in water. Both feet ... heavy ... like stones ... calves and knees ... heavy ... sinking ... deeper ... thighs and hips ... very heavy ... like lead ... Abdomen, chest, and back ... gravity pulling you down ... deeper ... Shoulders, arms, and palms ... very, very heavy ... Feel your entire head ... heavy like a stone ... Give your body completely and totally to the omni-present field of gravity. *(Pause.)*

Now experience your whole body heavy like a rock ... feel your whole body sinking ... deeper and deeper ... totally let go ... into the pull of gravity ... sinking deeper into stillness and silent awareness. *(Pause.)*

Now shift your attention as each part of the body is named, let all the heaviness drain away ... Let your body be buoyant and light, like a fluffy cloud ... Both feet ... limp and light ... calves and knees ... empty and free ... Feel it ... Thighs and hips ... hollow ... weightless ... Abdomen, chest, and back ... light and empty ... Shoulders, arms, and palms ... floating ... Head ... hollow ... empty. *(Pause.)*

Feel your whole body; empty ... light and hollow ... Sense the emptiness of your body, and silence of your mind. *(Pause.)*

Integration: Resting in Third Eye Awareness

Bring your attention to the center between your eyebrows and drop into the deepest level of relaxation. Here, there remains nothing to do or achieve, you have entered the domain of grace ... Allow yourself to merge into this space and be empty ...

In this domain of integration, you are witness of all that is happening but doing nothing to make it happen ... All that can never be done by your doing can happen only in the non-doing Presence of your being ...

Feel completely safe and comfortable as you hand yourself over to the power and protection of the Presence ... feel it ... experience it ... be it ... Hand over all fear, apprehension, and anxiety about all that you want to change, control, and manage ... let go of all doing ... Feel yourself as time-transcendent Presence, right now. *(Pause for 8 breaths.)*

Intention

Here your intentions are actualized and fulfilled with effortless ease. If you have self-defeating patterns or habits that are holding you back that you want to be freed from, make that your intention now... Repeat your intention now silently three times as words, an image, or felt sense. *(Pause.)*

Allow this intention to go to the deepest levels of recognition with no hesitation... Know that your higher Self recognizes, honors, and accepts your intention... Have faith and trust that it has been heard and is being acted upon by a higher power of the Source within... There is no need for you to do anything about it. *(Pause.)*

Affirmations

Allow your entire Self to respond spontaneously and effortlessly to focus on up to three of the following affirmations, choosing the ones that feel appropriate, here and now:

- I am released from my self-image to experience the infinite potential unfolding from within me...
- My Source is silent stillness. I rest in peace...
- I am the non-participative observer, separate from my thoughts and emotions that come and go...
- I hold no one responsible for all that has happened in the past. I am free and clear of all that has happened in the past...
- I go to the Source within that heals all conflicts and restores my health and peace of mind...
- I am at peace with myself as I am, and the world as it is...
- I return to the innate wisdom of my body to heal itself. I remain in restful awareness...
- I relax so completely and let go so fully that the inner healing blueprint of my body functions freely and optimally...
- I have entered a complete state of synergy and balance...

- I let the radiant light of love melt and disperse the blocks in my body and mind ...
- I replace resentment and regret with total acceptance and forgiveness ...

Higher Self and Spiritual Guide

Establish yourself firmly in faith and trust to receive the grace, protection, and guidance of the higher Self within you ... The more often you go to your Source, the easier it will be to return there and the longer you can stay there.

Feel the presence of your own spiritual guides, family members, or mentors surrounding you and blessing you ... accept their blessing and grace ... embody it and spread it wherever you go. (Pause.)

Now you have prepared the base from which you can carry out interactions with life and interpersonal relationships with the integrative power of love and the Source within ... You are the emissary of light and love ... carry it everywhere you go and to everyone you meet.

If you have an area that you feel needs healing—physical, mental, or emotional—allow this light and love to flow into that area now. (Pause.)

Closing and Externalizing

Now, begin to become aware of the rising and falling of the breath ... Slowly, feel yourself beginning to rise to the surface of awareness. (Pause.)

Sense the body resting on the floor ... the quality of the air as it touches the skin. (Pause.)

Gradually, you can move, as if you are waking from a restful sleep. (Pause.)

Bend your knees and pull them closer to your chest ... rock sideways gently ... take your time ... do not hurry.

Then just turn onto your side and curl into a fetal position ... Feel the safety, comfort, and protection of the womb of existence. (Pause.)

Bring your intention into your awareness again. Change nothing ... every time you find yourself in reaction, you are empowered to replace it with your intention. (Pause.)

Now you can gradually move and begin to sit up with your eyes closed. Continue to stay deep in this profound inner experience.

Regardless of what you consciously recognize that has or has not changed, know that something deep within has shifted to connect you with your intention.

Become aware of your body … and bring a deep sense of peace and content-ment with you as you bring attention back to the body. *(Pause.)*

Notice how relaxed the body is … how soft the breath is … how silent the mind is … how quiet the heartbeat is … Be still … and be grateful. *(Pause.)*

Know that you can easily enter here again and again.

Now, you may gradually open your eyes.

Kamini Desai, PhD is the author of *Yoga Nidra: The Art of Transformational Sleep,* and developer of the *I AM Yoga Nidra* app. She is the executive director of the Amrit Yoga Institute and an internationally recognized educator and developer of I AM Yoga Nidra immersions and professional trainings. Visit kaminidesai.com and amrityoga.org for more.

Resources

This script was originally written and created by yogi Amrit Desai. With per-mission, it is reprinted here and in *Yoga Nidra: The Art of Transformational Sleep* by Kamini Desai.

Books

Desai, Kamini. *Yoga Nidra: The Art of Transformational Sleep.* Twin Lakes, WI. Lotus, 2017.

Trainings

I AM Yoga Nidra Professional Training: https://amrityoga.org/upcoming-all/upcoming-yoga-nidra/

I AM Yoga Nidra Advanced Trainings: https://amrityoga.org/yoga-nidra/

Websites

kaminidesai.com

amrityoga.org

"Teachings of Kamini Desai (playlist)": https://www.youtube.com/playlist?list=PLwRuUO74cZ_tLYt904TnvuL0d4gijMUVg

Apps

Transformational Sleep App: https://www.kaminidesai.com/transformation-al-sleep-app

I AM Yoga Nidra App, 2018

Yoga Nidra for Restoring and Enhancing Health and Well-Being

Julie Lusk

Time: 20–30 minutes (Instructions are given to condense or expand the script)

Summary: This is for anyone who wants to optimize their health or is recovering from an illness or injury. Autogenic training, healing affirmations coupled with breathwork, and guided imagery for remembering well-being and enhancing cellular health and immunity are used. Your body will learn to quickly respond to health-enhancing suggestions. This is also helpful for improving skill-based performance (athletes, musicians, etc.) by learning how to calm the nerves on demand with verbal cuing.

The goal of autogenic training is to learn to stop the stress reaction and bring about the relaxation response. This is done by silently repeating phrases for feeling calm, heavy, and warm three to six times. Either use the instructions given for repeating both the heavy and warm statements or for either heaviness or warmth. This technique continues by combining phrases for feeling calm with breath awareness.

With diligent practice (three months or so) saying, "I am calm," will give fast physiologic results. In a meta-analysis of clinical outcome studies by Stetter and Kupper, autogenic training was shown to help treat tension headaches and migraines, mild-to-moderate essential hypertension (high blood pressure), coronary heart disease, asthma, pain management, anxiety disorders, mild-to-moderate depression and dysthymia, and functional sleep disorders.[24] Autogenic training has positive effects on mood, cognitive performance, and quality of life.

---

24. Friedhelm Stetter and Sirko Kupper, "Autogenic Training: A Meta-Analysis of Clinical Outcome Studies," *Applied Psychophysiology and Biofeedback* 27, no. 1 (March 2002): 45–98, https://doi.org/10.1023/a:1014576505223.

Guided imagination is also used for health: past, present, and future. This technique is endorsed by Herbert Benson, MD, the Harvard professor who identified the relaxation response. Research on the Benson-Henry Protocol (ten minutes of relaxation and eight to ten minutes of visualizing remembering wellness) yields beneficial clinical results in 60–90 percent of diseases.[25] An inner wisdom source is next invited to give insights followed by a time of being present.

Additional Notes: These techniques can be used in conjunction with proper medical care, not as a replacement. Wash your hands before starting since you will be covering your eyes with your palms during the meditation. Feel free to use the floor, sofa, bed, or chair if you are recovering from an illness or injury. Refer to chapter two for suggestions on using props, alternate positions, and for coping with special needs like back issues and other health conditions. Feeling supported physically enhances your experience by eliminating distractions in advance.

Stages	Process / Techniques
Preparation and settling in	Savasana
Sankalpa	Affirmation for healing and calming are embedded into the experience
Physical: Anna-maya kosha	Autogenic training focusing on heavy sensations followed by warm sensations
Energetic: Prana-maya kosha	Healing affirmations with breathing calmly
Mental: Mano-maya kosha	Guided imagery for healing and well-being for improving immunity, healthy cell renewal, and heart health. Imagery is used for remembering wellness

25. Herbert Benson and Richard Friedman, "Harnessing the Power of the Placebo Effect and Renaming It 'Remembered Wellness,'" *Annual Review of Medicine* 47 (February 1996): 193–199, https://www.ncbi.nlm.nih.gov/pubmed/8712773.

Stages	Process / Techniques
Intuitive: Vijnana-maya kosha	Intuitive guidance to support health using imagery
Bliss: Ananda-maya kosha	Joyful rest
True Self: Atman	True nature awareness
Sankalpa	Heartfelt pledge
Reawakening and closing	

Preparation and Settling In

Take time to get comfortable on the floor, bed, or in a chair. Remove your glasses. If your hands are clean, start rubbing your palms up and down against each other. That's right, keep it up, feeling your hands warming up. After they're nice and warm, place your palms over your closed eyes … allowing your eyes to be soothed by the darkness and the warmth … resting your eyes more and more … notice … Go ahead and rub or brush off your eyes and forehead for a while … and bring your hands down to your sides.

Align your head, neck, and back for good brain-body communication. Relax your shoulders down and away from your ears … Have your arms out to your sides with your palms gently turned up … let your fingers soften into relaxation … Adjust your body and any props so your low back, hips, legs, and feet feel supported. Please have your legs uncrossed and a comfortable distance apart. *(Pause.)*

Settle in, more and more. Feel free to make any adjustments to eliminate distractions in advance to lower the need to change positions later. If you do become uncomfortable, notice the sensations first, wait for the discomfort to clear, and then move with awareness if need be. Know that you're still benefitting when your attention drifts in and out or even if you fall asleep. This is your experience, so let it be customized for your optimal health and well-being.

Take a nice big breath in through your nose and sigh it out through your mouth … Do this a few more times at your own pace. *(Pause.)* Move your mouth and jaw all around, releasing tension … and bring your mouth to rest.

Remind yourself that it's time to relax into meditation and not for sleeping … Feel free to make movements or adjust your clothing for comfort.

Autogenic Training

Next, you will be given statements to silently repeat. There's no need to analyze or try to make anything happen, just listen and repeat. You can bring your attention back whenever distractions arise.

Heavy

Bring your attention to your right leg. Gently but firmly, press your leg down into whatever surface it's on … feel it … and release, letting go … Please silently repeat after me: *"My right leg is getting heavy … my right leg is getting heavier and heavier … my right leg is very heavy … my right leg is very, very heavy … I am really calm …"* And let it happen, feeling the heaviness in your right leg and relaxing more and more, heavier and heavier. If it helps, imagine it being weighted down.

Move your attention to your left leg. Press it gently but firmly into the surface supporting it … feel it … and release, letting go … Please repeat silently, *"My left leg is getting heavy … my left leg is getting heavier and heavier … my left leg is very heavy … my left leg is very, very heavy … I am really calm …"* And let it happen, relaxing more and more … feeling the heaviness in your left leg.

Take your attention to your right arm. Press it down … feel it … and release … *"My right arm is getting heavy … my right arm is getting heavier and heavier … my right arm is very heavy … my right arm is very, very heavy … I am really calm …"* Let it happen, feeling the heaviness in your arm, sinking into relaxation more and more.

Take your attention to your left arm. Press it down … feel it … and release … *"My left arm is getting heavy … my left arm is getting heavier and heavier … my left arm is very heavy … my left arm is very, very heavy … I am really calm …"* Let it happen, feeling the heaviness in your arms, sensing into relaxing more and more.

"My whole body is getting heavier and heavier … my body is very heavy … my body is very, very heavy … I am really calm …" Relaxing more and more. And let it happen, feeling the sensations in your whole body. There's no need to try and make anything happen. Perhaps noticing the earth's magnetic pull and sinking

into it ... perhaps feeling still and quiet ... And if at any time you notice that your body starts feeling light and buoyant, let it happen. Simply noticing your experience.

Keep bringing your attention back if unnecessary distractions arise. Remind yourself in your own way to remain alert, awake, and present. *(Pause.)*

Warm

Have your attention on your right leg ... Silently repeat after me, *"My right leg is getting warm ... my right leg is getting warmer and warmer ... my right leg is very warm ... my right leg is very, very warm ... I am really calm ..."* Softening into relaxation, more and more, warmer and warmer ... and let it happen, feeling the warmth in your right leg. If it helps, sense feeling your leg baking in the hot sunshine.

With your attention on the left leg. *"My left leg is getting warm ... my left leg is getting warmer and warmer ... my left leg is very warm ... feeling the warmth in your left leg ... my left leg is very, very warm ... I am really calm ..."* Sensing relaxation more and more, warmer and warmer, letting it happen as if the sun is warming it right up.

"My right arm is getting warm ... my right arm is getting warmer and warmer ... my right arm is very warm ... my right arm is very, very warm ... I am really calm. ..." Relaxing more and more, warmer and warmer, and it's happening.

"My left arm is getting warm ... my left arm is getting warmer and warmer ... my left arm is very warm ... my left arm is very, very warm ... I am really calm. ..." Relaxing more and more, warmer and warmer, and it's happening.

"My whole body is getting warmer and warmer ... my whole body is very warm ... my body is very, very warm ... I am really calm ..." Sensing relaxation, more and more. Letting it happen without trying, feeling the sensations in your whole body ... And if at any time you notice that your body starts feeling light and buoyant, light as a feather, let it happen. Simply noticing your experience.

Keep bringing your attention back if unnecessary distractions arise. Remind yourself in your own way to remain alert, awake, and present. *(Pause.)*

Healing Affirmations with Breathing Calmly

Silently repeating, *"My breathing is calm ... my breathing is calm ... my breathing is calm ... My breathing is smooth ... my breathing is smooth ... my breathing is smooth ... My breathing is calm and smooth ... my breathing is calm and smooth ... my breathing is calm and smooth ... I am really calm ... I am relaxing more and more ... I am really calm ... really calm ... relaxed and calm."*

Repeating to yourself, *"My immunity is just right ... my immunity is just right ... my immunity is not too much or too little ... my immunity is just right ... my immunity is just right ... my immunity is not too much or too little ... my immunity is just right ... I am really calm ... My cells are on track for health."*

Cells are constantly dissolving, repairing, renewing, and doing their work for optimizing health and well-being. Imagine all the cells that are at the end of their life cycle dissolving and being carried safely away ... uninvited cells, such as bacteria or unwelcome viruses, are disappearing ... cells that are no longer needed are dissolving now and being taken care of ... Imagine cells repairing and renewing ... Imagine the cells rebuilding ... cells are repairing and renewing and rebuilding ... Imagine cells maintaining and sustaining themselves for the right amount of time ... taking care of all your body's functions ... taking care of your heart ... taking care of your vital organs ... taking care of your glands ... taking care of all your body's functions ... Cells come to the end of their natural life cycle, dissolving ... renewing ... rebuilding ... functioning just right ... *"I am really calm."*

Either use any of these phrases or a healing phrase of your own during this long pause. *(Pause 1 minute.)*

Guided Imagination for Healing and Well-Being

It's time to awaken your mind's eye, your imagination. It's fine to see pictures and images, get a concept, or to use your other senses like feeling, hearing, touch, or smell. Naturally using your imagination in your own way.

Remember a time when you felt healthy and well, a time when your energy was good, feeling right with the world. It's fine to pretend by imagining what it would be like if it's hard to remember ... Take time to relive that experience by remembering what you were doing. Perhaps you were outside on a beautiful day. Possibly singing or dancing, playing sports, or were with friends, just so it's a moment in time when you felt healthy and well and doing whatever you enjoy. Imagine being there now and how it felt... having plenty of energy, stamina, and enjoyment. Bring it alive by using as many of your senses as you can by reliving what it was like, just like it's happening now... reliving it here and now... and in the present time.

And sensing it more and more, sensing into any feelings and bodily sensations... notice if there's any emotions, thoughts, or images that might naturally show up... and sensing into them. (Pause.)

Where do you notice well-being showing up in your body?... Showing up as physical sensation in the body... perhaps checking in with your chest... your breath... your arms and legs... around your face... sensing inside yourself, just for now, feelings of health and well-being. (Pause.)

And now, feeling full of health and energy in a future time. If you're recovering, imagine it all better and living fully again... seeing, sensing, being in the future brimming with health, vitality... imagining yourself enjoying the things you love, with plenty of health and well-being... feeling, sensing, seeing it now. (A ten-minute pause for remembering wellness is ideal.)

Intuitive Guidance

Sensing yourself right here and now and in the present moment. If you wish, imagine walking down a path of health and well-being... sensing being on your path. And as you're on your path, you notice being drawn to an offshoot... sensing yourself taking the offshoot... and noticing, sensing up ahead, a source of wisdom. It could be a person, an image, an animal, an impression, just so it's a source of wisdom that knows you deeply and always has your best interest at heart...

And if you wish, bringing this source of wisdom fully alive, more and more... allowing yourself to receive something, perhaps a message to guide you toward more health and well-being... Perhaps there's something to do to support your health. (Pause about 10 seconds.) Perhaps there's something to stop doing. (Pause about 10 seconds.) Sensing whatever people and circumstances are already in place to support you. (Pause about 10 seconds.) Sensing whatever people and circumstances are needed for support. (Pause about 10 seconds.) Sensing yourself with all the support and health needed for being on your path of meaning and purpose. *(Pause.)* Opening up to receive messages from this wisdom source. *(Pause about 30 seconds.)*

Joyful Rest

And letting all this go, just for now ... perhaps sensing having well-being ... perhaps sensing an inner place of peace and joy, unconditional peace and joy, where all is well. Soaking in the stillness and quiet during this long, silent pause. *(Pause 1–2 minutes or more.)*

True Nature Awareness

And now sensing an intrinsic dimension that is unconditionally healthy, well ... feeling connected ... wholeness. Resting in pure, unlimited awareness and oneness during this long, quiet pause. *(Pause 1–2 minutes or more.)*

Heartfelt Pledge

This is the time for your heartfelt pledge, your sankalpa, to appear, your heartfelt pledge to support a life of meaning and well-being ... letting it flow into your awareness, taking shape, more and more ... Perhaps it appears as a word or phrase or an image ... maybe it's formless ... perhaps letting it sing from your heart and soul ...

Imagining how it looks and sounds and feels ... allowing it to take shape in your life, more and more. *(Pause.)*

Reawakening and Closing

It's time to transition back, bringing with you all the insights and understandings you've received, for your sake, and for the sake of others. So, with this greater awareness of yourself, begin breathing more deeply, feeling the breath beginning to awaken you ... feeling your breath coming and going, infusing you.

It's time to stretch your body in ways that come naturally ... moving your arms and legs, and moving everything else ... Notice the movements, the physical sensations as you're stretching. *(Pause.)*

If you're lying down, please roll to your side and curl up ... Eventually, use your arms for support to press yourself up to sitting. *(Pause.)* Settle comfortably into sitting. *(Pause.)* Rest your hands on your lap ...

To seal this in and maintain the connection, touch the tips of the thumb and index fingers together. *(Pause.)* When you're ready, start blinking your eyes until they're fully open. Sensing your surroundings ... being aware of sounds ... being aware. *(Pause.)* Begin stretching about, awakening more and more.

With diligent practice of autogenic training, you will be skillful at using the verbal cue, *"I am calm"* to become calm. Remember to follow your intuitive guidance for better health and well-being.

Peace, peace, peace. (Om shanti, shanti, shanti.)

Yoga Nidra and Self-Healing
California College of Ayurveda

Contributed by Marc Halpern

Time: 40–45 minutes

Summary: The California College of Ayurveda Yoga Nidra emphasizes the understanding that Yoga Nidra is a state of consciousness and not a technique. It is a state of being conscious and awake while the body is deeply resting. From this state of consciousness, an individual can engage their sankalpa or "intention." The Yoga Nidra state of consciousness acts as a magnifier of intention, supporting a person's vision of themselves to manifest into reality.

Two sankalpas are established during this practice. The first occurs at the start of practice. This sankalpa is simply to stay awake and aware throughout the practice. The deeper sankalpa occurs toward the end of the practice through visualization. Having entered the state of Yoga Nidra, the practitioner visualizes themselves as they would like to be: healthy.

Stages	Process / Techniques
Preparation and settling in	Savasana
Sankalpa	Intention given to stay awake and aware
Physical: Anna-maya kosha	Tension release with mindfulness
Energetic: Prana-maya kosha	Personal exploration of prana (life force)
Mental: Mano-maya kosha	Healing guided visualization
Intuitive: Vijnana-maya kosha	Implied experience
Bliss: Ananda-maya kosha	Blissful awareness
True Self: Atman	Witnessing

Stages	Process / Techniques
Sankalpa	Visualization of healing statements
Reawakening and closing	

Preparation and Settling In

It's time to prepare your props ... Lie on your back, aligning your head, neck, and spine ... have your arms out to the sides with your palms up ... situate your entire back from top to bottom ... have your legs straight out, a comfortable distance apart ... make personal adjustments to your body and props for maximum comfort.

Sankalpa Setting

Go ahead and take a deep breath in and let it all out ... The next time you take another breath in, go ahead and give a deep sigh and say, "Aaah." Beautiful.

Now let's begin by establishing an intention to remain awake and aware for the entire practice. *(If alone, say these statements silently or out loud. If in a group setting, repeat them together after the instructor.)* "I will remain awake and aware." *(Pause.)* "Awake and aware."

It's time to completely relax. There is nowhere you need to go and nothing that you need to do for a while. Listen to my voice and allow my voice to guide your awareness. If you hear any outside sounds, let them take you deeper within. All the while, remember to stay 100 percent awake and 100 percent aware. Awake and aware.

Tension Release with Mindfulness

Let's relax the *hands, arms, and shoulders*. Go ahead and bring your awareness to your right hand. Notice your hand. Notice where it is and what it is touching ... Now bring your awareness to your right thumb. Notice if it is suspended in the air or if it is touching anything. Let go of any holding, control, or tension in your right thumb and let gravity take your thumb into whatever position that gravity wants it to be in. Letting go, letting go, letting go ... Now bring your awareness to the other four fingers of your right hand. Say hello to each finger and as you do, let go of any holding, control, or tension in each of the four fingers. Letting go, letting go, letting go ... Now bring your awareness to your palm. Notice the part of your palm that is closest to your little finger. Notice the part that is closest to your thumb. Let go of any holding, control, or tension in your palm and go deeper within. Deeper into relaxation. Deeper into surrender. Letting go.

Now bring your awareness to your wrist. Notice the top of your wrist that is facing the ceiling. Notice the bottom of your wrist that is touching the floor. Notice anything that is touching your wrist. Now bring your awareness inside of your wrist and with your mind's eye, look around. Notice if there are any areas of holding, control, or tension, and let them go. Allow your wrist to completely relax, and as you do, your palm and fingers become even more relaxed. Letting go, letting go, letting go. Deeper and deeper into relaxation. Deeper and deeper into surrender. *(Pause 10 seconds.)*

Now bring your awareness to the elbow. Notice the part that is facing the ceiling. Notice the part that is touching the floor. Explore your elbow with your inner eye. Notice if there are any areas of holding, control, or tension within the elbow or the muscles and tendons that surround it, and let them go. As you do, the forearm relaxes, the wrist surrenders more deeply. The palm becomes softer, and gravity takes your fingers wherever gravity wants them to be. Letting go, letting go, letting go. Deeper and deeper into relaxation, deeper and deeper into surrender. Letting go, letting go, letting go. *(Pause 10 seconds.)*

Now bring your attention to your left hand... notice your hand. Notice where it is and what it is touching... Now bring your awareness to your left thumb. Notice if it is suspended in the air or if it is touching anything. Let go of any holding, control, or tension in your left thumb and let gravity take your thumb into whatever position that gravity wants it to be in. Letting go, letting go, letting go... Now bring your awareness to the other four fingers of your left hand. Say hello to each finger and as you do, let go of any holding, control, or tension in each of the four fingers. Letting go, letting go, letting go... Now bring your awareness to your palm. Notice the part of your palm that is closest to your little finger. Notice the part that is closest to your thumb. Let go of any holding, control, or tension in your palm and go deeper within. Deeper into relaxation. Deeper into surrender. Letting go.

Now, bring your awareness to your wrist. Notice the top of your wrist that is facing the ceiling. Notice the bottom of your wrist that is touching the floor. Notice anything that is touching your wrist. Now bring your awareness inside of your wrist and with your mind's eye, look around. Notice if there are any areas of holding, control, or tension, and let them go. Allow your wrist to completely relax, and as you do, your palm and fingers become even more relaxed. Letting go, letting go, letting go. Deeper and deeper into relaxation. Deeper and deeper into surrender. *(Pause 10 seconds.)*

Now bring your awareness to the elbow. Notice the part that is facing the ceiling. Notice the part that is touching the floor. Explore your elbow with your inner eye. Notice if there are any areas of holding, control, or tension within the elbow or the muscles and tendons that surround it, and let them go. As you do, the forearm relaxes, the wrist surrenders more deeply. The palm becomes softer, and gravity takes your fingers wherever gravity wants them to be. Letting go, letting go, letting go. Deeper and deeper into relaxation, deeper and deeper into surrender. Letting go, letting go, letting go. *(Pause 10 seconds.)*

Now bring your awareness to the backs of both of your shoulders. Allow your shoulders to completely relax. Let go of any holding, control, or tension in the backs of your shoulders. As you do, your arms become even heavier and sink into the surface below. Letting go, letting go, letting go. *(Pause 10 seconds.)*

Now bring your awareness to the pits of your arms. Notice the four walls of each of your armpits. Let go of any areas of holding, control, or tension and go deeper within. Deeper and deeper into relaxation, deeper and deeper into surrender.

Your arms are now like two branches of a tree that have fallen to the ground. No longer attached, they lay by your side, still and at peace. Letting go, letting go, letting go.

Let's relax the *feet and legs.* Now bring your awareness to the toes on both of your feet. Say hello to each of the ten toes and let go of any holding, control, or tension … Now move your awareness to the soles of your feet. Let go of any holding, control, or tension in the soles of your feet … now bringing your awareness to the heels of your feet and your ankles. Notice the position of your feet. Let go of any holding, control, or tension in your ankles and let gravity take your feet wherever gravity wants them to be. Letting go, letting go, letting go. Deeper and deeper into relaxation, deeper and deeper into surrender.

Bringing your awareness to your knees. Notice the backs of your knees. Explore the area with your inner eye. Notice if there are any areas of holding, control, or tension in the backs of your knees and let them go. As you do, the calves and the ankles relax more fully, and the feet fall into whatever position is naturally right. Letting go, letting go, letting go.

Moving your awareness to the kneecaps. Notice the tops of the kneecaps that attach to your thighs. Notice the bottoms that attach to your shins. Let go of any holding, control, or tension in your kneecaps. Letting go, letting go, letting go.

Now bring your awareness to the tops of your thighs between the knees and your hips. Let go of any holding, control, or tension in the tops of your thighs and allow your legs to become heavier. Letting go, letting go, letting go … Now bring your attention to your inner thigh from your knees to your pubic bone. Let go of any holding, control, or tension in your inner thighs and surrender your legs more fully. Letting go, letting go, letting go … Now bring your attention to the back of your thighs. Notice the sensation of your thighs against the surface below you. Explore the bottoms of your thighs for any areas of holding, control, or tension and let them go. Allow your legs to become heavier and to sink into the surface below you. Deeper and deeper into relaxation, deeper and deeper into awareness.

And now bring your awareness to your buttocks. Let go of any holding, control, or tension in your buttocks. As you do, your thighs, knees, calves, and feet surrender even more. Letting go, letting go, letting go.

Your legs and feet are now like two more branches of a tree that have fallen to the ground. No longer attached, they lay by your side, still and at peace. Letting go.

Let's relax the *trunk* of the body. Now bring your awareness to your pelvis. Notice the sensation of your clothes against your skin. If you are covered by a blanket, can you feel it? … Now notice the muscles below your skin and allow them to relax. Go deeper still and, using your inner eye, look inside your pelvis. Let go of any holding, control, or tension in the organs of your pelvis. You don't have to know the anatomy, just look around and see if you can notice any areas of holding, control, or tension and let them go. Allow the life energy to flow freely without obstruction. Letting go, letting go, letting go. Deeper and deeper into relaxation, deeper and deeper into surrender. Letting go, letting go, letting go.

And now bring your awareness to your lower back. Let go of any holding, control, or tension in the muscles of your lower back. Now bring your awareness inside your lower back to the bones, the vertebrae. Allow them to completely relax. Letting go, letting go, letting go. Deeper into relaxation, deeper into awareness. Letting go.

And now, bring your awareness to your abdomen. Notice the sensation of your clothes against your skin. Go deeper and notice the layer of muscles below the skin and allow the muscles to relax. Go deeper still and look inside your abdomen. Notice if there are areas of holding, control, or tension inside of your abdomen. Allow the organs to completely relax. Letting go, letting go, letting go. Deeper and deeper into relaxation, deeper and deeper into surrender. Letting go, letting go, letting go.

Now bring your awareness to the areas between your shoulder blades. Allow the muscles of your upper back to completely relax. Let go of any holding, control, or tension in the muscles of your back. As you do, your entire body becomes heavier and sinks into the surface below you. Letting go, letting go, letting go.

And now, bring your awareness to your chest. Notice the sensation of your clothing against your skin. Now bring your awareness to the soft tissue of your breasts. Let go of any holding, control, or tension in the soft tissue of your breasts and let prana, the life energy, flow freely. Letting go, letting go, letting go ... Now bring your awareness to the ribs and notice the small muscles between your ribs. Let go of any holding, control, or tension in the small muscles between your ribs and go deeper within. Deeper into relaxation, deeper into surrender. Letting go. Now bring your awareness deeper still into your lungs. Let go of any holding, control, or tension in your lungs and allow prana, the life energy, to flow freely. Letting go, letting go, letting go. Deeper and deeper into relaxation, deeper and deeper into surrender. Letting go, letting go, letting go.

Now bring your awareness to the very center of your chest. Become aware of your heart. Let go of any holding, control, or tension in your physical heart. Let the prana, the life energy, flow freely through your heart and all the vessels within and surrounding it ... Now bring your awareness to your emotional heart. Let go of any holding, control, or tension in your emotional heart and let the prana flow freely, bringing healing to your deepest emotions ... Now bring your awareness to your spiritual heart and feel your connection to the Divine heart. Allow the love of the Divine to fill your heart. Let it overflow and circulate throughout your entire body. Visualize, sensing the love surrounding every cell … Now visualize, sensing it entering every cell. Let every cell of your body know that is it loved and it is love. Letting go, letting go, letting go. Deeper and deeper into relaxation, deeper and deeper into surrender. Letting go. *(Pause.)*

Let's relax the face and head. Now bring your awareness to your lips. Notice the top lip. Notice the bottom lip. Let go of any holding, control, or tension in your lips and allow all expression to be removed from your face. Your face is soft and at peace. Letting go, letting go, letting go.

Now bring your awareness to your jaw. Let go of any holding, control, or tension in your lower jaw. Let gravity take your jaw wherever gravity wants it to be. When your jaw is completely relaxed, gravity may slightly separate your lips and teeth. Letting go, letting go, letting go.

Bringing your awareness to your eyes, allow your eyelids to become so heavy that you could not open them even if you tried … Now bring your awareness deep inside of the sockets of your eyes. Let go of any holding, control, or tension in the small muscles deep inside. Letting go, letting go, letting go. Deeper and deeper into relaxation, deeper and deeper into awareness.

Now bring your awareness to the back of your head and your neck. Let go of any holding, control, or tension in the back of your head and your neck. As you do, let gravity take your head wherever gravity wants it to be. Letting go, letting go, letting go. Deeper and deeper into relaxation. Deeper and deeper into surrender. *(Pause 15 seconds.)*

Now bring your awareness to the crown of your head. Simply hold your awareness here and feel your connection to the Greater Whole … Allow the Divine light to enter and flow from above and down toward your hands and your toes. Visualize, sensing the light surrounding every cell of your body. Now allow the light to enter into each cell. Every cell of your body is now radiating with Divine light. Every cell is remembering its true nature as Spirit. You are remembering your true nature as Spirit, perfect and peaceful. *(Pause 30 seconds.)*

Now, expanding your awareness to include your *entire body* … your arms, your legs, your head, and your torso. Let go of any remaining holding, control, or tension and double your level of relaxation, allowing your body to become twice as heavy, to surrender twice as deeply … Your body is like an onion. Peel off another layer of holding, control, and tension and go deeper within. At the very center of your being is a body of light and energy. Allow the prana to flow more freely, all the while remaining 100 percent awake and 100 percent aware.

Awake and aware…letting go, letting go, letting go. Deeper and deeper into relaxation, deeper and deeper into surrender. *(Pause 30 seconds.)*

Personally Exploring Prana

And now take some time to explore your body on your own. If there is an area of your body that is in need of healing, this is a good time to give extra attention to that part, letting go of any remaining holding, control, or tension. Let the prana flow freely into those tissues. Letting go, letting go, letting go. Deeper and deeper into relaxation. Deeper and deeper into surrender. Letting go. *(Pause 45 seconds.)*

Healing Guided Visualization

And now in this deep state of relaxed awareness, create the ideal picture of yourself. See yourself completely healthy, completely whole…physically, emotionally, and spiritually. See yourself performing any activity that challenges you. See yourself living life without limitation. Know that your body and mind are perfectly healthy. Letting go, letting to, letting go. *(Pause 30 seconds.)* Awake and aware, awake and aware. *(Pause 30 seconds.)*

Blissful Awareness

And now, let go of your visualization. Know that it is being taken care of by the Divine and being supported to manifest. Take some time now to simply enjoy the bliss of Yoga Nidra. Enjoy the peace and joy that you are. Know that the core of your being is perfect and that your body and mind are healing. *(Pause 30 seconds.)* Not this body, not this mind…Not this body, not this mind. *(Pause 30 seconds.)*

Reawakening and Reinforcing the Healing Sankalpa

And now, as I count backwards from 10 down to 0, you will slowly begin to return awareness to your physical body, to present time and present space. There is no need to hurry. The count will be very slow. Even after the count is complete, you'll have plenty of time to make the transition. There is still nowhere you need to go and nothing you need to do for a while. *(Pause 10 seconds after each statement.)*

10. Remembering your true nature as Spirit.

9. Knowing that every cell of your body is surrounded by love. Every cell is love.

8. Knowing the light of pure awareness radiates from every cell of your body.

7. Knowing that prana is flowing freely through your body and that healing is taking place right now.

6. Knowing that the healing that is taking place right now will continue to occur even after this practice is complete.

5. Knowing that you can return to the state of Yoga Nidra at any time.

4. Taking with you into every day the relaxation and well-being that you are now experiencing.

3. Not this body, not this mind.

2. Consciousness and joy incarnate, bliss of the blissful am I.

1. Now go ahead and gently open and close your fingers . . . Go ahead and lick your lips.

0. Now go ahead and slowly turn your ankles in and out, side to side.

At your own pace and when you feel ready, go ahead and roll to your side and slowly return to a sitting position. There is still no hurry. Take your time. When you are sitting up, if there is a glass of water nearby, go ahead and take several sips. Sit quietly until you are ready to engage the world.

May the light of the Divine Healer illumine your heart and your mind, and may you always know that you are well.

Om shanti, shanti, shanti. (Peace, peace, peace.) Namaste.

Marc Halpern, D.C., CAS, PKS, is the founder and president of the California College of Ayurveda, the author of the popular book *Healing Your Life: Lessons on the Path of Ayurveda,* and the author of the mediation CD *Yoga Nidra and Self Healing.* He developed Yoga Nidra and Self-Healing from his experience utilizing Yoga Nidra as a tool for his own healing. In 1987, he was crippled with Lyme disease and cross immune reactions. He was introduced to the basic practice by Mary Richards, a teacher and psychologist. He practiced Yoga Nidra three times per day for an hour for seven years in order to facilitate his healing. During this time, he transcended the need for a script entirely and could simply lay down and enter the state. He's been teaching Yoga Nidra since 1990 and over the past twenty years modified the technique to match his experience to maximize the effectiveness of the practice. Visit ayurvedacollege.com.

_____

Resources

Healing Your Life: Lessons on the Path of Ayurveda. Twin Lakes, WI: Lotus Press, 2012.

Yoga Nidra and Self Healing CD

Website
www.ayurvedacollege.com

Healing Chakra Chorus
(Divine Sleep® Yoga Nidra)

Contributed by Jennifer Reis

Time: 25 minutes

Summary: This beautiful journey takes you into the depths of the chakra wheels or energy vortexes. There are said to be seven major highway intersections in the body where the three dominant energy channels, called ida, pingala, and sushumna, meet. Each of these seven intersections results in a chakra wheel. Each chakra represents a specific aspect of human nature and development such as receptivity, confidence, and inner wisdom. More information on the chakras is in appendix 2.

This practice guides you to become aware of each unique chakra through breath, color, and nature images. Guidance is given to imagine placing a healing flower on the many healing marma energy points on the body. Marmas are smaller wheels of energy throughout the body residing on the energy channels. To access deeper levels of internal health and well-being, the vibrational healing sound of aum (om) is potently "chanted" by healing flowers.

This is generally grounding and calming, develops the inner connection with body, breath, and energy, as well as the mind and emotions. It can help balance the endocrine system and hormones and can relieve insomnia and pain.

Stages	Process / Techniques
Preparation and settling in	Savasana
Sankalpa	Heart's intention
Physical: Anna-maya kosha	Body sensing with rotation of consciousness
Energetic: Prana-maya kosha	Breath awareness

Stages	Process / Techniques
Mental: Mano-maya kosha	Energy and sensory awareness with chakra energy visualization. Imaginary flowers are placed at healing points throughout the body with sound (nyasa)
Intuitive: Vijnana-maya kosha	Implied experience
Bliss: Ananda-maya kosha	Implied experience
True Self: Atman	Implied experience
Sankalpa	Heart's intention
Reawakening and closing	

Preparation and Settling In

Lie down on the floor or sit in a comfortable position. Feel yourself close to the earth. Take a deep breath in and, as you exhale, relax your whole body down toward the floor or chair ... allow earth to hold and support you now ...

Heart's Intention

Go deep inside to notice your heart's deepest longing. What does your heart desire? *(Give 30 seconds of silence.)*

Now create an intention based on your heart's longing. This is a positive statement in the present tense, as though it's already happening. State it three times to yourself. It is indeed the truth. *(Give 30 seconds of silence.)*

Body Sensing with Rotation of Consciousness

Begin to let your mind become very focused now on an inner journey through your body. Begin with the mouth. Feel lips ... notice inside of your mouth ... feel inside of mouth alive with sensation ... notice your nose ... breath ... Become aware of your ears: right ear ... left ear ... both ears ... ear canals ... and inner ears ... notice your ears receiving sound ... Feel your eyes: left eye ... right eye ... both eyes together ... feel your eyes glowing ... Notice the crown found at the top of the head ... Throat.

Feel the palm of the right hand ... thumb ... first finger ... second finger ... third finger ... fourth finger ... all five fingers ... aware of the whole right hand ... Wrist ... forearm ... elbow ... upper arm ... shoulder ... Notice the base of the throat. Now feel the palm of the left hand ... thumb ... first finger ... second finger ... third finger ... fourth finger ... All five fingers ... aware of the whole left hand ... Wrist ... forearm ... elbow ... upper arm ... shoulder ... throat. Notice the chest ... heart center ... abdomen ... solar plexus just below the ribs ... pelvis ... navel ... right hip ... thigh ... knee ... lower leg ... ankle ... foot ... toes ... and sole of right foot ... Feel again the pelvis ... left hip ... thigh ... knee ... lower leg ... ankle ... foot ... toes ... and sole of left foot. *(Slow the pace down.)*

Feel your root center between your sitting bones ... navel center ... solar plexus ... heart center ... throat center ... mouth ... third eye between the brows ... crown ... center back of the head ... neck ... between shoulder blades ... mid-back ... sacrum and low back ... root center.

In your mind, say, "I am awake and aware."

Breath, Energy, and Sensory Awareness with Chakra Visualization

Notice your natural breath ... Feel your breath washing through you, as though your inner body was a river flowing with breath ... Bring awareness to your root center between the sitting bones. And as you naturally inhale, feel your root filling with the color red. Vibrant red ... as you exhale it softens and liquefies ... Each inhalation, the root expands with red energy ... Imagine a tree with deep roots. *(Pause.)*

Now imagine a river of blue crystal water flowing through the central axis of your body—through your spine it flows from your root center between your sitting bones all the way up to the crown of your head ... Notice it flowing upward with your breath ... Now sense the blue crystal water flowing specifically from your root center up to the navel center. *(Pause.)*

As you next inhale, orange energy expands in your navel center ... as you next exhale, the navel softens ... as you inhale, orange energy flows wider in concentric circles ... Imagine an orange sunset. *(Pause.)*

River of blue flows from navel upward to solar plexus just below the ribs ... As you next inhale, feel your solar plexus expand with golden light ...

softens as you exhale... As you inhale like the sun itself, solar plexus shining yellow light... Imagine a golden sunflower. *(Pause.)*

Follow the flow of the stream from solar plexus up to your heart center... As you next inhale, emerald green healing energy expands your heart center... And each time you exhale, heart softens... gleaming emerald energy glows in heart center... Imagine a six-pointed star. *(Pause.)*

River flows your awareness from your heart up to the throat center... Now as you next inhale, spacious sky blue fills your throat center... As you exhale, throat naturally softens... Inhale healing sky blue energy expands the throat... As you exhale, the throat rests... Inhale, sky blue opens, wide and free, in the throat... Imagine here a happy blue butterfly. *(Pause.)*

River flows from throat up between the brows to third eye... luminous indigo energy fills your third eye as you inhale... And as you naturally exhale it relaxes... Inhaling, third eye energy expands... As you next exhale, third eye descends deeper into your being... Imagine a downward pointing violet triangle. *(Pause.)*

Blue river flows from the third eye up to crown of the head... crystal white light expands outward with each natural inhalation... With exhalation, crown softens... As you naturally inhale, crown expands with crystal light... As you exhale, the crown shines light up into the universe... Imagine a thousand petaled lotus flower. *(Pause.)*

Feel all these sacred energy centers come into perfect balance and harmony... These energy centers correlate to the glands and nerve plexuses in the physical body. Experience now the glands, endocrine, and nervous systems in perfect health and equilibrium. *(Pause.)*

In your mind, say, "I am awake and aware. Awake and aware in Divine Sleep."

Healing Nyasa Placement of Healing Flowers with Sound

Imagine a flower, any flower that comes into your awareness... perhaps noticing its shape, color, size... aware of the flower's texture and fragrance... Look right in its center and notice the color. Is there a shape or symbol here in the flower's center?... This sacred flower emanates healing nectar. *(Pause.)*

Now, you may like to place this flower at sacred healing points along the energy channels... First, place this flower in the palms and the backs of the hands...and in your wrists...Put this flower in the centers of your fore-arms...in the elbow joints...in the centers of the upper arms...Lay this flower in the shoulder joints...Set flowers on the soles and tops of your feet...in the ankle joints...mid-calves and shins...Flowers in the knee joints...Rest flowers at the centers of your thighs, front and back...in the hip joints.

Set three flowers on the sacrum or low back, forming a triangle...Place a row of flowers on the vertebrae all the way up to where the spine meets the skull...Place a flower on your crown...Rest two flowers on your eyes...and one on your third eye...Lay a row of flowers from the notch in the throat down the front midline to the pubic bone.

Now hear the sound of aum (om) emanating from each flower, simultaneously...As you inhale, the flowers brighten...As you exhale, they sound aum...Inhale, they become brilliant...Exhale, they stream the sound of aum. *(Pause.)*

The flowers join together in a chorus of aums, healing and refreshing you on all levels...Now rest here for some time receiving all the restoration you need. *(Give two minutes or so of silence.)*

Heart's Intention

Remember now your intention...repeat it in your mind and heart a few times. *(Give 30 seconds of silence.)*

Reawakening and Closing

Become aware of sacred centers and channels in the body...Notice your body's innate ability to heal itself...Sense the facets of your wisdom and perception that you will use to bridge this vision of healing in your everyday life...Become aware of your thoughts and feelings as you feel yourself supported by the earth...

Feel the breath...Breathe more deeply...feel breath in the fingers and begin to move your fingers to the rhythm of your breath...Feel the earth holding and supporting your body...Roll over to one side...use your arms to lift yourself up to sitting...Sitting now, integrating and absorbing your experience. *(Give 30 seconds of silence.)*

You have abundant light, peace, health, and well-being.

Peace, peace, eternal peace.

When you're ready, you may open your eyes.

Jennifer Reis, E-RYT 500, C-IAYT, Kripalu Schools of Yoga and Integrative Yoga Therapy faculty, creates sacred space for students to journey into realms of deep peace and healing. An authentic and spirited leader, Jennifer has been teaching for more than twenty-two years and is the creator of Divine Sleep Yoga Nidra and Five Element Yoga. Her CD, *Divine Sleep Yoga Nidra,* is the best-selling CD in the Kripalu Shop. Visit jenniferreisyoga.com for more.

Resources

Audios

Recorded version of "Healing Chakra Chorus" and others are available at jenniferreisyoga.com

Training

Divine Sleep Yoga Nidra Teacher Training—40-hour certificate training; Yoga Alliance YACEP, Kripalu 1000 Hour Teacher Training, Social Workers, and others.

Bihar Yoga Nidra:
Intermediate Chakra Visualization

Contributed by Swami Shankardev Saraswati

Time: 20–30 minutes depending on speed of instruction and time left for visualization

Summary: This is an intermediate stage Yoga Nidra practice from the Bihar Yoga (Satyananda) tradition. It is a dharana (concentration) practice and part of a series of Yoga Nidra techniques that gradually unfold an authentic experience of the chakras and the psychic body, the vijnana-maya kosha. It starts the process of purifying the subtle body and awakening the chakras into consciousness. It is preparation for a deeper dive into the chakras and the subtle body. Once you can visualize the simple forms of the chakras outlined here, then more complex visualizations are added, including symbols and mantras. See appendix 2 for more information about the chakras, their pronunciation, and their symbols.

To prepare, one must be able to relax and remove exhaustion from the body through the process of pratyahara (deep relaxation), otherwise it is not possible to hold the symbol in the field of consciousness, resulting in sleep instead. Old emotional patterns can surface in people who have not done initial training in purification through meditation.

Stages	Process / Techniques
Preparation and settling in	Savasana and spontaneous breath awareness
Sankalpa	Resolve
Physical: Anna-maya kosha	Rotation of consciousness

Stages	Process / Techniques
Energetic: Prana-maya kosha	Breath awareness focused on the third eye and naval centers
Mental: Mano-maya kosha	Chakra visualization
Intuitive: Vijnana-maya kosha	Implied experience
Bliss: Ananda-maya kosha	Implied experience
True Self: Atman	Implied experience
Sankalpa	Resolve
Reawakening and closing	

Preparation and Settling In

Lie on the floor with your feet comfortably apart. The backs of your arms are touching the floor, your chin is slightly tucked in to gently lengthen your neck and align it with your spine... Relax your whole physical body... Each time you exhale, let go of a little more tension from your body... Aim to be comfortable so that during the practice of Yoga Nidra you do not have to move your physical body. Make any adjustments now so that you do not need to move later.

Remember that two things are important in the practice of Yoga Nidra... The first is no movement... and the second is no sleeping... Aim to remain awake and aware throughout the practice of Yoga Nidra.

Spontaneous Breath Awareness

Become aware of your natural, spontaneous breath. Be aware that your breath is moving into and out of the body... without any effort... Your breath and your awareness are moving together. Notice which part of your body moves first as you breathe in... and which moves first as you breathe out. *(Pause.)*

Remain aware of each and every breath. Do not become lost in any thoughts. Do not sleep. Aim to remain awake and aware throughout the practice of Yoga Nidra. *(Pause.)*

Resolve

Now remember your sankalpa, your resolve. The sankalpa is a short, positive statement that summarizes your intention and resolve to achieve something great in your life. If you do not have a sankalpa, contemplate something now that you would like to achieve, so that you can use the practice of Yoga Nidra to improve yourself and your life. Once you have your sankalpa clearly and firmly in your mind, repeat it three times with total focus and sincerity, knowing that you are planting your sankalpa deep into your subconscious mind where it will continue to empower you to achieve your sankalpa, even while you are asleep. Remember that anything in life can fail you but not the sankalpa made during the practice of Yoga Nidra. *(Pause.)*

Rotation of Consciousness

You are now going to rotate your awareness through the parts of your body. As I name a part, take your awareness to that part. Remain relaxed, still, and aware of each and every part that I name.

Rotation of consciousness through the parts of the body starts at the right thumb. Take your awareness to your right thumb, second finger, third finger, fourth finger, little finger, all five right fingers at once. Right palm, back of the right hand, wrist, forearm, elbow, upper arm, shoulder, armpit, side, waist, hip, buttock, thigh, hamstrings, knee, calf, ankle, heel, sole. Right big toe, second toe, third toe, fourth toe, fifth toe, all five toes at once. *(Pause.)*

Take your awareness to the left side of your body ... to the left thumb, second finger, third finger, fourth finger, fifth finger, all five left fingers at once. The left palm, back of the left hand, wrist, forearm, elbow, upper arm, shoulder, armpit, side, waist, hip, buttock, thigh, hamstrings, knee, calf, ankle, heel, sole. Left big toe, second toe, third, fourth, fifth, all five toes at once. *(Pause.)*

Moving your awareness up the back of the body, become aware of the backs of both legs. Right buttock, left buttock, both buttocks. Right shoulder blade, left shoulder blade, both shoulder blades. The whole right side of the back, the whole left side of the back, both sides of the back as one. Whole spinal cord, whole spinal cord, whole spinal cord. *(Pause.)*

Back of the neck, back of the head, top of the head, forehead, right eyebrow, left eyebrow. The eyebrow center, eyebrow center, eyebrow center ... Right eye, left eye, both eyes. Right ear, left ear, both ears. Right cheek, left cheek, both cheeks. Right nostril, left nostril, the whole nose. Upper lip, lower lip, both lips ... lower jaw. Throat ... right collarbone, left collarbone, both. Right chest, left chest, both sides. Heart center, heart center, heart center ... Upper part of the abdomen ... lower part of the abdomen ... the whole abdomen, navel center ... pelvic floor. *(Pause.)*

The whole right side of the body ... the whole left side of the body ... the right and left sides of the body as one. The whole back of the body ... the whole front of the body ... the back and front of the body as one ... The whole physical body, whole physical body, whole physical body. *(Pause.)*

Breath Awareness Focused on the Third Eye and Naval Center

Now become aware of the breath moving up and down the two nostrils ... As you inhale, the breath moves from the nose tip up toward a point between the two eyebrows ... This point is a trigger point for the third eye, anja chakra, in the center of the brain. Follow the breath with your awareness for a few moments. *(Pause.)*

Take your awareness to the navel center and observe the navel moving up as you inhale and down as you exhale. The navel is a trigger point for the manipura chakra in the spinal cord. Imagine that as you inhale, the breath is moving into the navel, and as you exhale the breath is moving out of the navel. Become aware of this movement of the breath into and out of the navel for a few moments. *(Pause.)*

Chakra Visualization

Take your awareness up and down the whole physical spine ... feel each and every part of the spinal cord. From the pelvic floor up along the back to the point in the middle of your head where the third eye is situated.

Now become aware of your whole spine from muladhara chakra at the base of your body, in the middle of the pelvic floor, up to ajna chakra, the third eye, which lies in the center of your head ... Become aware of each and every part of the spine at the same time ... the whole spinal cord ... Be aware of every part of the spine from muladhara chakra up to ajna chakra. *(Pause.)*

Take your awareness to the pelvic floor and feel a point of luminous, radiant energy vibrating in its center ... Visualize the muladhara chakra in the form of a dark red lotus flower with four petals ... Become aware of the powerfully uplifting vital energy vibrating in the center of this lotus. *(Pause.)*

Take your awareness to the sacrum and feel a point of luminous, radiant energy in its center ... Visualize the swadhisthana chakra as a vermilion colored lotus with six bright red petals . . . Become aware of the potent life-giving energy vibrating in the center of this lotus. *(Pause.)*

Take your awareness to the point of energy in the spine behind the navel and feel a point of luminous, radiant energy vibrating there . . . Visualize the ten yellow petals of the manipura chakra lotus . . . Become aware of the transformational power vibrating in the center of this lotus. *(Pause.)*

Take your awareness to a point of energy in the spine behind the breastbone and feel a point of luminous, radiant energy vibrating there . . . Visualize the twelve blue petals of the anahata chakra lotus . . . Become aware of the loving, compassionate energy vibrating in this lotus. *(Pause.)*

Take your awareness to a point of energy in the spine behind the throat pit and feel a point of luminous, radiant energy vibrating there . . . Visualize the sixteen purple petals of the vishuddhi chakra lotus . . . Become aware of the powerfully purifying energy vibrating in this lotus. *(Pause.)*

Take your awareness to a point of energy in the center of the head behind the eyebrow center and feel a point of luminous, radiant energy vibrating there . . . Visualize the two silvery gray petals of the ajna chakra lotus . . . Within the lotus is an om sign . . . Become aware of the powerful energy that underlies and supports your conscious mind vibrating as the mantra "om" in this lotus. *(Pause.)*

Above the ajna chakra, at the top back of the head, is the bindu. Bindu is the mystic point that divides the constantly changing mundane world from the eternally unchanging transcendent reality. Visualize a bright full moon. Become aware of this point and contemplate its meaning. *(Pause.)*

Hovering just above the head is the thousand petal lotus at sahasrara. It is composed of infinite light, which spreads in all directions. It has no energy and is composed of pure consciousness. *(Pause.)*

You are now going to descend back down through the chakras. Become aware of the bindu and its symbol, the moon. Take your awareness to ajna chakra and the two silvery gray petals . . . to vishuddhi chakra with sixteen purple petals . . . anahata chakra with twelve blue petals . . . manipura chakra with ten yellow petals . . . swadhisthana with six bright red petals . . . muladhara with four dark red petals.

You are now going to ascend and descend through the chakras. Feel the qualities of all the chakras as you ascend and descend and whatever sensations are emanating from them.

Take your awareness down to muladhara ... ascend to swadhisthana ... ascend to manipura ... ascend to anahata ... ascend to vishuddhi ... ascend to ajna ... ascend to bindu ... ascend to sahasrara. *(Pause.)*

Now descend from sahasrara ... descend to bindu ... descend to ajna ... descend to vishuddhi ... descend to anahata ... descend to manipura ... descend to swadhisthana ... descend to muladhara. *(Pause.)*

Resolve

Now remember your resolve, your sankalpa. Repeat your sankalpa three times with awareness and great resolve, knowing that anything in life can fail you but not the sankalpa made during the practice of Yoga Nidra.

Reawakening and Closing

And now become aware of your physical body lying in savasana, the corpse pose, practicing Yoga Nidra ... Notice how you feel as a result of this practice of Yoga Nidra. *(Pause.)*

Gradually take your awareness outwards into the room in which you are lying and become aware of your physical environment ... Slowly move your fingers and toes ... When you are fully back and grounded in your body, sit up. The practice is over.

Dr. Swami Shankardev Saraswati is a Western medical doctor, Yoga Acharya (Master of Yoga), Yoga therapist, author, and teacher. He lived and trained for ten years with Swami Satyananda at the Bihar School of Yoga from 1974 to 1985. He now teaches online, including courses on Yoga Nidra, at bigshakti.com.

Resources

Website
www.bigshakti.com

Sleep Well with Yoga Nidra

Julie Lusk

Time: 30 minutes

Summary: This practice is different from traditional Yoga Nidra. Normally, Yoga Nidra is like being asleep but with the added benefit of remaining alert and aware. The intention here is to help you fall into regular sleep. Practicing this will release physical, emotional, and mental tensions to clear the decks for a good night's rest. This enables you to begin drifting from being awake into becoming drowsy and getting sleepier until you doze off into sleep.

Sleeping and dreaming are very natural and valuable. Your body and mind already know how to sleep and to benefit from dreams. However, many of us get off track and struggle with going to sleep and staying asleep. Yoga Nidra can reset your system so restful sleep can happen, providing you the benefits derived from the natural sleep cycles of lightly dozing, sleeping deeply, and dreaming too.

We all have nights when we feel half awake and half asleep, and other nights when the body is asleep but we feel awake emotionally or mentally. This practice can help by flushing out bodymind stress, so remnants and concerns don't follow us into sleep. If you should awaken before it is time, this gives you solutions to use instead of stressing out. You will be able to drift easily back to sleep by using the skills provided here for help in riding the ups and downs of sleeping, or simply enjoy resting in the beauty of the night.

Establish and use a routine at bedtime so you can get the seven to nine hours of sleep needed nightly for restoring your health and energy. Go to bed and get up at roughly the same time, even on weekends. Turn down the lights; the darker, the better. Unplug your devices and set aside whatever might distract you from sleeping. Going to sleep takes about twenty minutes for most people. There is no need to feel rushed.

Feel free to go along with this meditation, as much or as little as you like, until you go to sleep. Change it to suit yourself. It's up to you.

Stages	Process / Techniques
Preparation and settling in	Savasana
Sankalpa	Heartfelt pledge
Physical: Anna-maya kosha	Sensory awareness, inner eye gazing (chidakasha), and rotation of consciousness
Energetic: Prana-maya kosha	Intentional breathing for relaxation
Mental: Mano-maya kosha	Mental and emotional brushing for clearing tension
Intuitive: Vijnana-maya kosha	Implied experience
Bliss: Ananda-maya kosha	Implied experience
True Self: Atman	Implied experience
Sankalpa	Heartfelt pledge
Closing	Falling asleep

Preparation, Settling In, and Heartfelt Pledge

Please give yourself permission to enjoy the process of Yoga Nidra awareness while you transition into dozing off and sink into deep sleep. Now is the time for slowing down to have a good night of rest with some sound sleep, knowing you'll wake up at the appropriate time, feeling restored and refreshed.

Get yourself comfy. You can be on your back, side, or stomach. In other words, however you like to go to sleep. *(Pause.)*

Close your eyes, like lowering the shades, nice and comfy... It's time for allowing your daytime awareness to gradually recede, like a turtle safely withdrawing into its shell, so nighttime and sleeping awareness can expand into sleeping soundly. Remembering just how special and important sleeping and dreaming are for your well-being. *(Pause.)*

It's time to cross the bridge from wakefulness into sleeping and dreaming, taking whatever time is needed for this. And as you're crossing this bridge, you can start to unload and clear away whatever you want... For instance, what's no longer needed that you might want to toss off the bridge...what might get in your way of having restful sleep and beneficial dreams?...Saying goodbye to these things, at least for now, so they won't bother your sleep.

Please take a big breath in and sigh it out. *(Pause.)*

And now, remembering what will help you feel protected and safe during the night...imagine being surrounded by whatever you would like to have around you that's reassuring for you...Perhaps there's people, animals, guardians, or special things, anything that's comforting and will support sleeping, imagining this now. *(Pause.)*

Perhaps, you may want to plant some seeds for having some helpful dreams, ones that have insights, dreams that are beneficial. And if you like, being able to remember them later on. *(Pause.)*

During this valuable transition, you're welcome to recall a few areas of your life you're grateful for. *(Pause.)*

How about tucking yourself in even better...Go ahead and stretch, if you wish...shift around to get more and more settled. Adjusting your covers and pillows to get even more comfortable and cozy. *(Pause.)*

Go ahead and remind yourself that it's time for sleeping through the night. Use your own words to ask for cooperation and support from your body, mind, and spirit for a good night's rest. *(Pause.)*

Let's continue moving through the process of going to sleep and enjoying the experience of Yoga Nidra, allowing your body to release tension and calming down any static into stillness. Enabling your mind to clear away thoughts that clutter up awareness, sweeping them away, while emotions fade into the background.

Sensory Awareness and Inner Eye Gazing (Chidakasha)

Feel free to yawn...just open your mouth up real wide, breathe in, in, in, and let yourself yawn. Go ahead and try it a few times...Open your mouth up real wide, breathe in, in, in, and let yourself yawn. *(Pause.)*

Next, please bring your attention to your mouth...moving your jaw up and down and all around...and now coming to rest...Perhaps moistening your lips...and letting the corners of your lips quiet down into softness...And pressing your tongue against the roof of your mouth, and letting it rest...So, softening your tongue, more and more, until it kind of hovers in there. There's no need for tension, softening your tongue relaxes the mind, all nice and quiet.

And taking your attention to your forehead. With your eyes closed, begin lifting and lowering your eyebrows... and letting them come to rest, smoothing out this entire area. *(Pause.)*

Even though your eyes are closed, you still have vision, inner vision. All that's needed is to gaze at the inside of your eyelids and softly toward the middle of the eyebrows, like watching a movie screen. It might look dark, there may be splotches of color, images, or glimmers of light. It doesn't matter what appears and disappears, it's about impartially watching whatever is coming and going... and each time your mind wanders, simply shift your attention back to gazing inside, simply softly gazing with quiet eyes. *(Longer pause.)*

Feel free to fall asleep anytime. *(Pause.)*

Let your hearing expand into listening off into the far distance, letting the sounds come and go without having to name them or react in any way... only listening to the distant sounds. *(Pause.)* And listening to the nearby sounds as they happen, simply letting the sounds be heard, plain and simple... And now letting the sounds blend, coming and going... And if distracting sounds should happen, allow them to help deepen your experience. Simply notice how it sounds and let it go, perhaps focusing on something else. *(Pause.)*

It's time to gently squeeze your hands into a ball, like a bud of a flower... and to slowly let your fingers unfold like a bud becomes a bloom... allowing your hands and fingers to rest comfortably, more and more.

Wiggle your toes... and let them rest.

You may yawn or take a big breath in... and sigh it out.

It's okay to go to sleep anytime. *(Pause.)*

Rotation of Consciousness

It's time to move your awareness throughout your body. Feel free to silently repeat each body part as it's named. You might enjoy getting a concept of it, or sense feeling it, or even picture it, whatever comes easiest for you... bringing restfulness all around as we go. There's no need to move at all, simply letting your mind's eye follow along from place to place, bringing restful sleep throughout your mind and body.

It's time to mentally find your right hand... sensing where your right hand is... and the right thumb... the pointer finger... the middle finger... the ring finger... and the baby finger... the palm of the hand... the back of the hand... the wrist... the elbow... right shoulder top... the armpit... down the right side to the hip... the knee... ankle... heel... bottom of the foot... top of the foot... the big toe... the second toe... the third toe... the fourth toe... and the baby toe... and now the whole foot... the whole entire foot.

And now, mentally find your left hand... sensing your left hand... the left thumb... the pointer finger... the middle finger... the ring finger... and the baby finger... the palm of the hand... the back of the hand... the wrist... the elbow... left shoulder top... the armpit... down the left side to the hip... the knee... ankle... and heel... the bottom of the foot... top of the foot... the big toe... the second toe... the third toe... the fourth toe... and the baby toe... and now the whole entire foot... having a direct experience of your whole foot.

If you get distracted, it's no big deal. Simply bring your attention back to whatever we're doing.

Moving your awareness now to the base of your spine... up to your lower back... mid-back... and upper back... to the top of your head.

And now to the right eyebrow... left eyebrow... between the eyebrows... right eyelid... left eyelid... feeling your eyelids getting heavier and heavier... right eyeball... left eyeball... and the line between your eyelids, the line between the eyelids... letting your eyes rest... gazing at the inside of your eyelids, watching whatever's happening. *(Pause.)*

And now the right ear... the left ear... right cheek... left cheek... the nose... and the tip of the nose... the upper lip... the lower lip... the line between the lips... and the corners of the lips... And now, going inside the mouth... sensing the inside of the mouth... Start pressing the tongue into the roof of your mouth or the back of your teeth... and letting your tongue rest, softening it, more and more... And now to the throat... the heart... the upper abdomen... the navel... the lower abdomen... and the base of the spine.

Becoming aware of the presence of your entire right leg, the whole of your right leg... and becoming aware of your entire left leg, the whole left leg... and now both legs at the same time, both legs... Now being aware of your right arm, the entire right arm, just for now... and the whole left arm, the entire left arm... and both arms at the same time... Moving now to the whole back side of your body, sensing the entire back side of your body...and now the front side, the entire front side...and both sides together, as one...Sensing your head...and face...and your head and face at the same time...Being aware now, of your whole self, your whole self.

You're welcome to move around for more comfort, shifting and adjusting your position, your covers, your clothes, for more comfort, so you can easily go to sleep, right when it's time for sleeping.

Breathing With an Intentional Exhalation and Effortless Inhalation

And now, bring your attention to your breathing. Breathing through your nose, using your mouth only to the amount it's needed. Begin to focus on your exhalation, focusing on breathing out, and letting the inhalation take care of itself...Following your exhalation out, again and again, as it naturally happens...Each time you naturally breathe out, you may begin to silently say, "going out" or simply "out." Silently saying "out" while breathing out for the next few minutes. *(Pause 1–2 minutes.)* And softening your tongue...and having quiet eyes...continuing to breathe as effortlessly as possible. Letting go, more and more and falling asleep anytime. *(Pause.)*

Mental and Emotional Brushing

How about feeling a wave of healing relaxation rinse through you? Allowing it to start at the top of your head, calming your mind, brushing away tension and unnecessary thoughts, and making room for soothing sleep and beneficial dreams...brushing and rinsing away emotions and feelings as it goes.

This wave of relaxation begins to wash down your neck and shoulders...continuing down your arms to your fingertips, rinsing away any thoughts or memories, emotions or feelings, making way for some pure awareness...Brushing away injuries and hurts, past or present...healing and restoring...and washing and rinsing all around the top of your torso...When you're ready, it goes all around your heart and lungs, gently removing what's no longer needed, clearing and cleansing...and on into all the other vital organs, rinsing and clearing and settling down into rest and restoration...and this wave of rest and relaxation, begins pouring in and around your hips, going all around your hips...and it's moving down your legs, taking away any thoughts and memories, and any feelings or emotions, just rinsing and brushing all the way down to your feet and toes. Washing tension completely and safely away... and now, you can use this technique wherever you might want to use it, to continue to cleanse and clear away distractions, leaving a sense of peacefulness inside. *(Pause.)*

Heartfelt Pledge

Into this potent place, you may make a personal pledge, reflecting something that supports your growth, a positive quality to support your personality, your actions, your spirit. Perhaps something that gives your life direction. *(Pause.)* Remembering your pledge when you wake up is a valuable way to start your day.

Closing

It's okay to drift off to sleep if you're ready and to cycle naturally through all the valuable levels of sleep, restoring your body, mind, and spirit. Otherwise, continue to let your breathing soothe you, more and more, like a lullaby, listening to it like a comforting song, dropping distracting thoughts and feeling into the stream of your breath to be carried away... softening your tongue, more and more... again and again. And having your eyes become very quiet, comforted by the cover and protection of the eyelids, softly gazing at the inside of the eyelids like watching a movie, knowing it's okay to either hover for a little longer on the edge of sleep, or to drop off into sleep... Sleep well.

Resources

Sleep Well: Yoga Nidra by Julie Lusk is available on CD, MP3, and for streaming. Additional tracks are included featuring soothing Native American style flute music and one of ocean waves. Visit JulieLusk.com, Amazon, iTunes, and other online outlets.

LifeForce Yoga Nidra Script for Calming Frazzled Nerves, Anxiety, and Easing Exhaustion

Contributed by Rose Kress

Time: 30 minutes

Summary: This Yoga Nidra comes from LifeForce Yoga, a style of Yoga developed for managing energy fluctuations to mood issues like depression, anxiety, and trauma. LifeForce Yoga emphasizes accessibility for all. It operates from the yogic understanding that there is no separation between you and the infinite. Every individual is whole and complete as they are. Any suffering comes from the mistaken belief of separation. From this understanding, stress, depression, anxiety, and trauma are viewed as constrictions rather than something that defines us. LifeForce Yoga seeks to empower people to discover their unique wholeness and cultivate ease. See "Lifting Depression and Energy with Life-Force Yoga Nidra" by Amy Weintraub for another application of the LifeForce method.

The Yoga Nidra practice presented here was created for people struggling with anxiety. It is also appropriate for people suffering from trauma. It is contraindicated for people with schizophrenia and other mental health conditions where there may be disassociation, as is true for all Yoga Nidra practice.

It can be difficult to concentrate when the mind is anxious and the nerves are frayed. Consider a physical Yoga practice, or some sort of movement, prior to this practice to burn off some energy prior to lying down. Going at a faster speed at the beginning of Yoga Nidra can help hold attention during the process.

Stages	Process / Techniques
Preparation and settling in	Savasana
Sankalpa	Heartfelt prayer and inner sanctuary
Physical: Anna-maya kosha	Rotation of consciousness
Energetic: Prana-maya kosha	Side-to-side breathing awareness
Mental: Mano-maya kosha	Awareness of opposites
Intuitive: Vijnana-maya kosha	Implied experience
Bliss: Ananda-maya kosha	Joy of love visualization
True Self: Atman	Implied experience
Sankalpa	Heartfelt prayer
Reawakening and closing	

Preparation and Settling In

Set yourself up so that the body can be comfortable for the duration of the practice. Placing a support, like a thin pillow, under the head invites the nervous system to relax. Placing a cushion under the knees helps to release tension in the low back. Feel free to use an eye pillow. Maybe even covering yourself up with a blanket as the body begins to cool. *(Pause.)*

During this practice of Yoga Nidra, we welcome everything—every sensation, every breath, feeling, emotion, thought, belief, even distractions—as pathways to a deeper experience of our wholeness. So, allow distractions and the wandering of the mind to be reminders to return to the practice and the present moment.

Feel the whole body lying on the floor... The whole body, breathing itself. Feel your body supported by the ground... Notice the ways in which your body softens into the support of the ground... Notice the ways in which your body does not soften... Take a moment here to adjust yourself so that you are ten, fifteen, maybe even twenty percent more comfortable so that you don't need to move, knowing that if you do need to move you have total permission to do so.

During this practice we will cultivate a sense of calm and stillness. Take a moment here to identify what the experience of being calm and still is for you... Perhaps it's a feeling in the body, maybe a memory, or perhaps an image arises. Welcome and breathe with your experience of calm and still. Invite the body and the mind to connect with calm and still... During the practice, as you hear the words, "calm and still," allow yourself to experience moments of calm and still. With practice, you will be able to recall calmness and stillness with ease. *(Pause.)*

Heartfelt Prayer

Begin to connect with your heart... As you breathe with your heart, invite a heartfelt prayer to arise. Your heartfelt prayer is that seed that your heart is planting for your personal growth, your spiritual well-being. It's what your heart is longing for more than anything else in this world for you. The heartfelt prayer is something that you are growing in your life. If it seems as though nothing is arising, the heart is offering up the prayer of stillness and receptivity. Take three deep breaths affirming this heartfelt prayer as though it is true and already happening... On your third exhale, let your heartfelt prayer go and remain open to the ways in which this prayer arises during the practice and your day. *(Pause.)*

Inner Sanctuary

Let's welcome and establish your inner sanctuary. The inner sanctuary is that place, real or imagined, that when you go there in your mind or in real life you feel peaceful, or serene, or at ease. Imagine yourself there now. It could be a place in nature, a special room, or a feeling in the body... There might even be beings present that support you on your journey. Imagine yourself in your inner sanctuary right now. Feel yourself becoming more peaceful, more serene, and more at ease... This inner sanctuary is available to you at any point during the practice or during your day when you feel that need for more peace, serenity, or ease.

Rotation of Consciousness

Bring the awareness back to the body... The whole body lying on the floor... The whole body breathing itself, in and out. The whole body, calm and still... There may be moments when the mind wanders during the practice. When that happens, anchor your mind on the sound of my voice and the present moment. As we move awareness through the body, sense and feel each part of the body from the inside. If it supports the practice and supports holding the attention, you might even wish to visualize that part of the body.

Sense the mouth. Roof of the mouth, floor of the mouth, sidewalls, left and right. Sense the tongue, the lips, and the lower jaw. Experience the entire mouth and lower jaw as calm and still... Sense the left ear. The hills and valleys of the outer left ear. The density of sensation in the inner left ear canal. Sense the right ear. Hills and valleys of the outer right ear. The density of sensation in the inner right ear canal. And now make the mind big. Big enough to experience both ears at the same time. Both ears, an experience of calm and stillness. *(Pause.)*

Completely focused, sense the tip of the nose. The breath moving in the left nostril... The breath moving in the right nostril... The breath moving in both nostrils at the same time... Sense the eyes. The left eye, eyebrow, temple, and cheekbone. The right eye, eyebrow, temple, and cheekbone. Again, make the mind big enough, expand the awareness to experience both eyes at the same time. Both eyes and an experience of calm and stillness... Sense the forehead, the scalp, back of the neck. The sides of the neck—left and right—and the throat. Experience the whole face, head, neck, and throat as calm and still...

Sensing the whole left side of the body lying on the floor. Whole left side of the body, calm and still... Sense the left shoulder, elbow, wrist, the left palm, and all the left fingers. Even becoming aware of the space between the left fingers. The calm and still energy between the left fingers... Back of the left hand, forearm, upper arm, and armpit. Experience the whole left arm as calm and still. Even becoming aware of the energy that surrounds the left arm. The calm and still energy around the left arm...

Sense the left side of the ribcage, front, side, and back. The gentle flow of breath moving in the left side of the rib cage... Sense the left side of the abdomen and low back. Experience the gentle flow of breath moving in the left side of the abdomen and low back...

Sense the left hip, knee, ankle, sole of the left foot, and all the left toes. Even becoming aware of the space between the left toes, the calm and still energy between the left toes... Top of the left foot, lower leg, thigh, and buttock. Experience the whole left leg as calm and still. The calm and still energy that surrounds the left leg... Sensing and experiencing the whole left side of the body as sensation. *(Pause.)*

Side-to-Side Breathing

And now imagine the breath traveling in through the sole of the left foot up the left side of the body all the way to the crown of the head. On the exhale, imagine the breath traveling from the crown of the head down through the right side of the body to the right foot... Inhaling through the left side of the body to the crown. Exhaling from the crown through the right side of the body to the right foot. Imagining every breath moving in through left and out through right... Inhaling left. Exhaling right. Awareness riding the breath in through the left and out through the right. Awareness riding the breath from the left side of the body to the right side of the body. *(Pause.)*

Pouring the awareness into the right side of the body. Let go of the breath. Sense and feel the whole right side of the body lying on the floor. The whole right side of the body, calm and still. *(Pause.)*

Rotation of Consciousness Continues

Sensing right shoulder, elbow, wrist, palm, and all the right fingers. Even becoming aware of the space between the right fingers. The calm and still energy between the right fingers... Back of the right hand, forearm, upper arm, and armpit. Experiencing the whole right arm as calm and still. The calm and still energy that surrounds the right arm. *(Pause.)*

Sense the right side of the ribcage, front, side, and back. The breath moving in the right side of the ribcage... Sense the right side of the abdomen and low back. The subtle sensations of breath moving in the right side of the abdomen. *(Pause.)*

Sensing right hip, knee, ankle, sole of the right foot, and all the right toes... Even becoming aware of the space between the right toes. The calm and still energy between the right toes... Top of the right foot, lower leg, thigh, and buttock. Experience the whole right leg as calm and still. Even becoming aware of the calm and still energy surrounding the right leg and the whole right side of the body. *(Pause.)*

The calm and still energy that surrounds the entire body. Expand the awareness to feel and experience the entire body as sensation, calm and still sensation. *(Pause.)*

And now sensing into awareness. The field of awareness in which these changing sensations rise and fall; in which these changing breaths rise and fall. In which the energy rises and falls and yet awareness remains unchanged ... Awareness remains constant, ever present. *(Pause.)*

Awareness of Opposites

Sensing back into the body, welcome an experience of grounding. Perhaps an experience where the body feels solid and connected to the earth. Welcome that experience of grounding, of steadiness ... Invite the whole body to experience grounding. The feet, the legs, grounded. The arms, the hands, grounded. The shoulders, grounded. The whole body grounded and connected to the earth ... Become absorbed in the experience of grounded.

And now welcome an opposite experience. The experience of brightness; of the body as bright and illuminated. The feet and legs experiencing brightness. The hands and arms experiencing brightness. The face bright. The whole body experiencing brightness, like a light is shining from the inside ... The whole body, bright.

And now shift the awareness back to the experience of grounding. The whole body grounding ... Sensing back into brightness. The whole body bright ... Now expand the awareness to hold grounding and brightness at the same time. That indescribable and undefinable experience of both at the same time ... Then sensing into the field of awareness itself, where these changing sensations of grounding and brightness rise and fall, and yet awareness remains constant. *(Pause.)*

Now welcome an area of discomfort in the physical body. Sense into a discomfort. Not necessarily the big one, but perhaps a numbness, an unpleasant sensation. Resist the urge to change anything about this discomfort, and instead, you're invited to fully experience discomfort ... Breathe with discomfort. Welcome discomfort. Allowing the full expression of discomfort. *(Pause.)*

Shift the awareness to an experience of comfort in the physical body. A comfort, maybe an awake-ness, a sense of ease in the physical body. Resist the urge to spread this comfort and instead simply experience comfort for comfort's sake ... Breathe with comfort in the physical body. Allow comfort. Experience comfort; the fullness of comfort in the physical body. *(Pause.)*

Sense back into discomfort ... This time sensing a little deeper into discomfort. And perhaps there's an emotion woven into the experience of discomfort in the physical body. No need to search or dig. Simply welcome any emotion that is present, woven into the experience of discomfort in the physical body. If no emotion is present, welcome this experience … Breathe with discomfort and any emotion that is present. *(Pause.)*

Shifting awareness back to comfort in the physical body … Sensing deeper into comfort in the physical body, perhaps there is an emotion woven into the experience of comfort in the physical body. Again, no need to dig. Simply welcoming any emotion that is present, woven into this experience of comfort in the physical body. If no emotion is present, welcome this experience … Breathe with comfort and emotion. *(Pause.)*

Sense back into discomfort and emotion … Sensing deeper into discomfort. Perhaps there is a belief woven into the experience of discomfort and emotion. Without searching, welcome any belief that is present. Allow a belief to arise. No need to search. And if no belief is arising, welcome this experience … Breathing with discomfort, emotion, and belief. Allowing the fullness of the experience of discomfort, emotion, and belief … Allowing discomfort, emotion, and belief to fully unfold within the field of awareness. *(Pause.)*

Sensing back into comfort … Sensing deeper into comfort and perhaps there is a belief woven into the experience of comfort and emotion. Without searching, welcome any belief that is woven into the experience of comfort and emotion. Allow a belief to arise. And if no belief is arising, welcome this experience … Breathing with comfort, emotion, and belief. Welcome the fullness of the experience of comfort, emotion, and belief … Allowing comfort to fully unfold within the field of awareness. *(Pause.)*

Stepping back now into the field of awareness in which discomfort and comfort rise and fall; in which emotions and beliefs rise and fall … Awareness holding all of these at the same time. And yet awareness is so much more. Always present, constant … Welcoming everything just as it is. *(Pause.)*

Joy of Love

Now diving into the heart space … Sense into the heart space beyond the physical heart. The heart space where love resides. The experience of love and the heart's true nature, which is to love unconditionally … Welcome this experience of love that holds everything. Invite this experience of love to begin to expand … This experience of unconditional love spreading through the rib cage, like a smile … This experience of unconditional love spreading into the hands, the fingertips, so that the hands and fingertips are operating in the world from a place of love and acceptance. *(Pause.)*

Invite this unconditional love to spread into the feet, the legs, so that the legs carry this body through the world with love and acceptance... Invite this unconditional love to expand to the lungs so that every breath is one of love and acceptance... Love and acceptance spreading into the head, the mind so that all the thoughts, the words that are spoken, can come from a place of love and acceptance. *(Pause.)*

This unconditional love filling the entire body. Your entire being filled with love, acceptance, and self-acceptance... If you wish, invite this unconditional love and acceptance to spread out beyond the boundaries of this physical body. Spreading out into the space that surrounds the body. Out to loved ones... out into the planet... out into every being that needs a little more love and acceptance... Let go of judgment and imagine that this unconditional love and acceptance touches the heart of every two-legged being, three-legged, four-legged, finned, and feathered creature. Every being. Even the beings with many legs. Every being. Even the beings with flower petals. With leaves and bark. The stones. Spreading this unconditional love and acceptance into every molecule of dirt. Every drop of water. Every molecule of air. *(Pause.)*

Imagine this whole planet surrounded and filled with unconditional love and acceptance... Experience and know yourself as a being that lives on this planet of unconditional love and acceptance. Feel yourself loved and accepted as you are. Welcome this experience from that field of awareness. Welcome everything just as it is. *(Pause.)*

Heartfelt Prayer and Closing

From this experience of welcoming everything just as it is, once more invite your heartfelt prayer... breathing with your heartfelt prayer. Imagine it as true and already happening. *(Pause.)*

Feel your body lying on the floor, calm and still... The body breathing itself. Join in with this natural rhythm of breath. Inviting it to deepen. As the breath is deepening, begin to sense into the space around you, hearing any sounds inside the room, outside the room, seeing any light behind the eyelids... Breathing even deeper now, begin to wiggle the toes, the ankles, the fingers, and the wrists. Beginning to stretch, to reach, to yawn yourself awake. *(Pause.)*

And then rolling yourself over to one side. *(Pause.)*

Give yourself the hug that you have been longing for. You deserve it. Offering yourself thoughts, words of love and acceptance at this moment... Using an exhale, press yourself into a seated position. *(Pause.)*

Let's seal in all the good aspects, all the freeing aspects of our practice of Yoga Nidra using the healing tone of Om.

Rose Kress, E-RYT-500, C-IAYT, is the owner and director of the LifeForce Yoga Healing Institute. She is a longtime Yoga practitioner, Yoga therapist, and trauma survivor. Through LifeForce Yoga, she found relief from anxiety and trauma. Rose is the creator of the popular Best Practices webinar series and has numerous Yoga Nidra recordings and videos. She travels internationally to lead the LifeForce Yoga Practitioner Training. Visit Yogafordepression.com for more.

Resources

Website

www.yogafordepression.com/store

Books

Kress, Rose. *Awakening Your Inner Radiance with LifeForce Yoga: Strategies for Coping with Stress, Depression, Anxiety, & Trauma.* Lebanon, Oregon: LifeForce Yoga, 2019.

Weintraub, Amy. *Yoga for Depression: A Compassionate Guide to Relieve Suffering Through Yoga.* New York: Broadway Books, 2004.

Weintraub, Amy. *Yoga Skills for Therapists: Effective Practices for Mood Management.* New York: W. W. Norton, 2012.

Lifting Depression and Energy
with LifeForce Yoga Nidra

Contributed by Amy Weintraub

Time: 30 minutes

Summary: This is designed to lift and sustain feelings of joy and can be used by anyone. However, it is especially valuable in times when a constricted mood state, like depression, becomes overwhelming. An ability to accept whatever mood is visiting—with the knowledge that it will change—increases and an improved sense of well-being and joy can be experienced. It is designed to help you on your journey to sustain optimum mental health and empower you when you have lost touch with who you truly are. LifeForce Yoga Nidra was used in a study where symptoms of depression, as measured on the Beck Depression Inventory, went from 30 down to 16.[26]

This is contraindicated for people with schizophrenia and other mental health conditions where there may be disassociation. This is true for all Yoga Nidra practice.

See *Calm Frazzled Nerves, Anxiety, and Ease Exhaustion with LifeForce Yoga Nidra* by Rose Kress for another application of the LifeForce approach.

Stages	Process / Techniques
Preparation and settling in	Savasana and tension release
Sankalpa	Heartfelt prayer
Physical: Anna-maya kosha	Rotation of consciousness

---

26. Sumedh Mankar, "Effects of Utilizing Yoga Nidra on Reducing Symptoms of Depression and Anxiety in a Psychiatric Population," *The Journal of the American Osteopathic Association* 112 no. 8 (2012): 543. Abstract C19.

Stages	Process / Techniques
Energetic: Prana-maya kosha	Breath awareness
Mental: Mano-maya kosha	Awareness of opposites
Intuitive: Vijnana-maya kosha	Witnessing
Bliss: Ananda-maya kosha	Welcoming and witnessing waves of joy with awareness of opposites
True Self: Atman	Dwelling
Sankalpa	Heartfelt prayer
Reawakening and closing	

Preparation and Settling In

You may wish to use a cushion or blanket under your knees, an eye pillow to cover your eyes, and a light cover for your body. A folded blanket under your head will tilt the chin forward slightly, supporting the mind to relax.

Come into savasana, lying on your back with your legs a comfortable distance apart, palms face up and chin slightly tucked.

Invite a deep breath in and hold it for a moment, tightening the glutes, tighten the face, make fists of the hands, and tighten as many muscles as you can, and let go … Inhale deeply again and tighten as much as you can. Squeeze whatever is no longer serving you, and then let it go. Release and let your body soften into the earth … Inhale deeply again and tighten as much as you can. Squeeze all the judgments, the self-limiting beliefs, the expectations, everything that is blocking the free flow of healing energy and love. Squeeze, squeeze, squeeze, and completely let go. Allow your body to soften into the earth. *(Pause.)*

Now join with your own natural rhythm of breath, welcoming the breath wherever it lands … letting it deepen … Ride the waves of your breath home to who you are inside, beneath the current mood, the social mask, the costumes you put on. Ride the waves of your breath home to the ground of your being where you are intimately and eternally connected, the ground of your being that knows no separation.

Heartfelt Prayer

From this place of wholeness, invite a heartfelt prayer to arise, revealing itself in your heart's mind. What's the burning bush in your heart? ... The seeds are already present in your life. When you've identified the seed of the longing, plant it in your heart, and say it to yourself in the present tense, as though it's already blossoming. For example, "Joy breathes through me now," or "A drop of joy flows through me now," or "I am open and available to give and receive love and joy." This is your sankalpa, your resolve.

Take four or so more natural breaths as you imagine breathing your sankalpa into your heart, letting the heart expand with each breath. Breathe your sankalpa through every cell. The beginning and end of your practice are the most fertile times to nourish the seed of your sankalpa. If you plant the sankalpa every day during Yoga Nidra, that seed will blossom more fully in your life.

Rotation of Consciousness and Breath Awareness

The whole body is lying on the floor. Become aware of the whole body, lying on the floor. A global awareness of sensation shimmering through and around the whole body lying on the floor.

During the practice of Yoga Nidra, the mind may subside for moments into sleep or into a spacious awareness without thought. Allow my voice to be an anchor, drawing you back to awareness of the present. Sense each body part as we move systematically, almost mechanically through the body, beginning with the mouth.

Sense deeply into the mouth ... sense the roof of the mouth and the floor of the mouth. Sense the tongue. Let the tongue fall away from the roof of the mouth. Inner left cheek, inner right cheek. Sense the lips, the sensation between the lips. Whole mouth, hollow and empty. Feel the hollow spaciousness of the mouth as shining, expansive sensation. All the structures of the mouth, hollow and empty.

Trace a line of sensation flowing from inside the mouth through the hollow tubes of the inner ear canals, all the way out to the hills and valleys of the outer ears. Left ear, right ear, hollow and empty. Sense the nose. Experience the hollow spaciousness inside each nostril. Left nostril ... right nostril ... hollow and empty.

Sense the eyes, those orbs of glowing sensation. Sensation in the eyes, all the way back into their cradles, feeling the structures around the eyes. Cheekbones; left ... right. Temples; left ... right. Eyebrows; left ... right. Bridge of the nose.

Upper eyelid, lower eyelid...space between the eyelids...spaces between the lashes. Left eye, right eye, still behind their lids.

Sense deeply into the big brow muscle in the middle of the forehead and trace a line from the midpoint of the brow back through the brain, deep into the primitive brain stem at the base of the brain. Moving forward and center to the amygdala, the hippocampus. Notice subtle sensation in the right hemisphere, the left hemisphere...Sense outward into the head...the whole head, from the crown of the head all the way to the back of the head. Notice the neck and the hollow space behind the neck. Sense into the throat, hollow and empty. The hollow notch at the base of the throat.

Breathe into the left side of the body. Whole left side of the body lying down. Follow the sensation in the left shoulder all the way down the arm to the empty spaciousness at the palm of the hand and all the little bones in the fingers. Left thumb, index finger, middle finger, ring finger, little finger. All the fingers at once. The spaces between the fingers, the energy around the whole left hand. Left wrist, elbow, and the hollow space of the armpit. Whole left arm lying on the floor. Feel the whole left arm lying on the floor.

Sense the left rib cage and the space between the left arm and the left rib cage. Sense the spaces between the ribs. Bottom left rib. The space between the bottom left rib and hip bone. Left kneecap, the hollow space behind the knee. Shin, ankle, all the way down to the hollow space at the sole of the foot and all the little bones in the toes. Big toe, second toe, third toe, fourth toe, fifth toe. All the toes simultaneously. The spaces between the toes.

Sensation flowing through the whole left side of the body. Whole left side of the body, spacious, hollow, and empty. Feel the whole left side of the body lying on the floor. The energy field shimmering, glowing around the left side of the body lying on the floor.

Inhale through the sole of the left foot, sensing the whole left side, all the way up to the crown of the head. Exhale down through the right side. The life-force energy of prana flowing as a circle of breath. Breathing up through the left side and down the right side, beginning to sense into the whole right side. Waves of breath, lapping against the right shore of your body. Invite four or so waves from left to right on your own. (Four breath pause.)

Sense the right side of the body, lying on the floor. Whole right side of the body lying on the floor. Sensation in the right shoulder, all the way down the arm to the hollow spaciousness at the palm and all the little bones in the fingers. Right thumb, index finger, middle finger, ring finger, little finger. All the fingers at once. Spaces between the fingers. Back of the hand. Right wrist, elbow, and the hollow space of the armpit. Whole right arm on the mat. Feel the whole right arm on the mat, glimmering with sensation.

Sense the right rib cage and the space between the right arm and the right rib cage. Sense the spaces between the ribs. Sense to the bottom right rib and the hipbone and the space between the bottom right rib and the hipbone... Sense the kneecap, and the hollow space behind the knee. Shin, ankle, all the way down to the hollow space at the sole of the foot and all the little bones in the toes. Big toe, second toe, third toe, fourth toe, fifth toe. All the toes simultaneously. The spaces between the toes.

Sensation flowing through the whole right side of the body. Whole right side of the body, spacious, hollow, and empty. Feel the whole right side of the body lying on the floor. The energy field glowing, shimmering around the right side of the body, lying on the floor.

Breathe into both sides of the body simultaneously. Become aware of both sides of the body. Awareness of the whole body lying on the floor. Whole body is lying on the floor.

Awareness of Opposites

Sense the whole body lying on the floor and the energy field expanding around the body.

Is there an area of discomfort in the body? Perhaps an unpleasant tightness or numbness. Allow the breath to join the area of discomfort without trying to change anything. Aware of discomfort in your body. Breathe into the area of discomfort.

Is there an area of comfort in the body? Perhaps a pleasant sensation of tingling or lightness. Let the breath join with the comfort in your body, without trying to change anything. Simply notice comfort in the body. Breathe into the area of comfort.

Can you flow back and forth between the area of discomfort in the body and the area of comfort in the body? Take two or so long breaths into the area of discomfort or constriction. *(Pause for two breaths.)* Take two or so long breaths into the area of comfort or freedom. *(Pause for two breaths.)*

Sense into the deeper awareness that welcomes discomfort and comfort, constriction and freedom...Sensing back now into a greater timeless awareness, expanded and spacious, aware of both discomfort in the body and comfort. Welcoming sensation.

Body at rest, waves of feeling arising. Allow waves to wash over and through. Perhaps a wave of grief...Perhaps a wave of sadness laps against the shores of this body, heavy, lying on the earth, grounded, heavy, sinking in the sand. No words necessary. No labels, just a felt sense of sadness or heaviness...Allowing the tide to rise with the emotion and recede.

Welcoming and Witnessing Waves of Joy with Awareness of Opposites—Bliss

From this earthbound heaviness, a lightness arising...Welcoming a wave of joy. Body light and floating. Perhaps a wave of love for no reason...No story...Joy for no reason. Body light...No words necessary. Allowing the tide of joy to rise and recede...Waves of bliss to wash over and through...Joy.

Allow the tides to move through you. Waves of sadness, washing over and through. *(Longer pause.)* Waves of joy washing over and through. *(Longer pause.)* High tide. Low tide...A storm at sea...A sunny beach...A clear, calm day, embracing the changing tide of emotions. *(Longer pause.)*

Embracing both the discomfort in the body and the unpleasant emotion, and the comfort in the body and the pleasant emotion...Can you sense back into a spacious awareness where discomfort and comfort, pleasant and unpleasant, heaviness and lightness can live in the bodymind?

Awareness expanding, formless...timeless. Here...Now...From the ground of your being, your own true nature, embracing the waves of life. Unsullied by whatever has happened to you. One with all that is. You are the ocean of bliss...ananda...bliss, welcoming it all.

Awareness of the energy around the body, bliss expanding and spacious like a great cosmic smile. Invite the smile to enter your heart. Maybe a memory comes—a moment of happiness. Inhale and breathe the moment around your heart. Heart smiling. Your eyes. Eyes smiling. Your cheeks. Cheeks smiling. Memory dissolves. Whole body smiling. Blissful smile extending beyond the limits of your physical body lying on the floor. Bliss expanding beyond the limits of this room. Bliss spacious and expanding beyond the limits of this country.

Bliss spacious, radiant, expanding beyond the limits of this planet. Bliss shimmering eternally, intimately.

No separation between the ocean of healing energy that surrounds you and the rivers of healing energy flowing through you now. From this expanded place of spacious awareness, everything you need is flowing through you now. Whole. Here. Now. No separation. *(Longer pause.)*

Heartfelt Prayer

Begin noticing your body lying on the floor... Notice the sounds in the room [name some sounds if you are leading a group]. Invite the breath to deepen and breathe into your wholeness... Breathe your heartfelt prayer, your sankalpa through every cell. Your sankalpa is already present, growing. Nourish the seed of your sankalpa with your breath and your attention. As you breathe your heartfelt intention through you, completing your Yoga Nidra practice, you are fertilizing the seed of intention that will manifest fully, blossoming in every facet of your life. *(Pause.)*

Reawakening and Closing

As you end your Yoga Nidra practice and return to your daily life, resolve to pause throughout your day to remember who you truly are, beneath your mood, beneath any label, beneath all the to-dos of your daily life. Simply pause and sense back into this greater awareness of who you are. Not separate. Whole.

Begin to stretch and move in your own way. Perhaps stretching arms overhead and taking in a breath that moves from toes to fingertips. Feel your energy. Your contentment. You may wish to bring your knees to your chest and give yourself a gentle rock from side to side... Roll onto one side. *(Pause.)* Before you rise, say something kind to yourself, just the way you would to a small animal or a little child in your care. Say something loving and understanding, maybe to a younger part of yourself that needed to hear it. *(Pause.)*

This is a practice, just like rolling out your mat. When you've said that kind thing, use your upper hand to press yourself into a seated position.

Namaste. Thank you for practicing Yoga Nidra with me today.

Amy Weintraub, MFA, E-RYT-500, YACEP, C-IAYT, is the founder of LifeForce Yoga and a pioneer in the field of Yoga and mental health. She is the author of *Yoga for Depression* (Broadway Books) and *Yoga Skills for Therapists* (W.W. Norton) and numerous articles, book chapters, and online audio-video practices. Visit amyweintraub.com for more.

Resources

Books

Yoga for Depression: A Compassionate Guide to Relieve Suffering Through Yoga. New York: Broadway Books, 2004.

Yoga Skills for Therapists: Effective Practices for Mood Management. New York: W. W. Norton, 2012.

Yoga for Your Mood Deck—Card deck. Boulder, CO: Sounds True, 2021.

Recordings

LifeForce Yoga Nidra to Manage Your Mood—CD

LifeForce Yoga to Beat the Blues—DVD

iRest Yoga Nidra Meditation
for Chronic Pain Relief

Contributed by Stephanie Lopez

Time: 30–45 minutes

Summary: This practice is offered to support those meeting acute or chronic pain. It is a variation of iRest Yoga Nidra meditation, comprising the 10-step protocol and introducing the use of color in the practice. It is open to anyone. Specifically, it may support those interested in pain relief, building emotional regulation, and promoting post-traumatic growth. Through using an inner resource, which is an unchanging felt sense of ground, security, and well-being, the iRest protocol is trauma sensitive, allowing practitioners to have choice and control over their experience. You may weave in the inner resource at any time during the practice—whether or not it is indicated in the script.

There are guiding principles underlying iRest that are useful in daily life and during meditation. Welcoming what is—no matter how challenging the sensation or circumstance—is foundational. To truly welcome, we need to embody a sense of nonjudgmental presence, curiosity, self-compassion, and patience. Rather than trying to fix or change pain, we are allowing it to be there and reveal its hidden layers.

This particular practice incorporates noting when we meet pain as pure sensation and peeling off the conceptual label which may otherwise bind us to our habitual pattern. We then explore the intensity of sensation non-conceptually. We also welcome emotions, beliefs, and images that may be present while interweaving the inner resource of well-being. We use the practice of working with opposites using color.

Color has been used as a traditional way to support healing in cultures worldwide. Taoist Yoga, Tibetan Yoga, Indian Yoga, and Western modalities have incorporated color symbolism as part of their meditation and scientific understanding. Combining color with breath and imagery supports the meditator to meet, and potentially move beyond, pain.

Regulation of the autonomic nervous system and building self-compassion is fostered. It enhances a sense of meaning and purpose in one's life. These are a few known factors that can help people living with pain. Regular practice enables you to meet each moment of your life with unshakable peace and well-being, no matter how challenging or difficult your situation.

Additional Notes: This is written for someone who is lying down. However, it can be done in a prone, side, sitting, or standing position.

Stages	Process / Techniques
Preparation and settling in	Savasana and welcoming messengers
Sankalpa	Intention for this practice Senses wide open Heartfelt desire Inner resource
Physical: Anna-maya kosha	Rotation of consciousness breath and energy awareness
Energetic: Prana-maya kosha	Breath awareness
Mental: Mano-maya kosha	Meeting pain with awareness of sensation, breath, energy, emotions, and cognitions
Intuitive: Vijnana-maya kosha	Welcoming and witnessing opposites; cognitions
Bliss: Ananda-maya kosha	Sheath of joy and equanimity
Pure I-ness: Asmita-maya kosha and Sahaj	Welcoming well-being, whatever is present
True Self: Atman	Everything just as it is
Sankalpa	Heartfelt desire
Reawakening and closing	Taking the practice into the world

Preparation and Settling In

Begin your practice of iRest Yoga Nidra in a comfortable position, arranging your body so you feel completely supported to enter a deep state of rest and self-inquiry. Allow your legs to be apart, arms away from your body, and palms turned upwards. Have support under the back of your head so that your chin remains below the level of your forehead throughout your practice to assist your thinking mind to relax. Support your back by placing a blanket under your knees or thighs. If helpful, place an eye bag over your eyes... If you could be five or ten percent more comfortable, make any adjustments to bring ease and well-being throughout your body and mind... Releasing the body into the support of the surface underneath it.

Welcoming Messengers

During iRest, welcome every experience as a messenger that's inviting you to explore particular sensations, emotions, and thoughts, or the recognition of being spacious awareness. Welcoming and responding to each messenger that arrives in your guesthouse of awareness with curiosity and openness... And setting everything free to be there, just as it is. *(Pause.)*

Sankalpa

Intention for this Practice

Note your intention for this practice... Perhaps to remain alert and attentive... Or to inquire into a particular intensity of sensation that you wish to work with today... Open to what is... perhaps abiding as joy, Being, or awareness... Fully welcoming and affirming your intention for today's practice with your entire body and mind. *(Pause.)*

Senses Wide Open

Now, welcome the space of the room around you... The sense of the body resting into the surface supporting you... Bring attention to your senses, allowing each perception to come to you... Sounds around and within your body... without grasping toward sound... The nose smelling... The mouth tasting... The inner eyes open to seeing... The touch of air on your skin... Sensations within your entire body... Sensing the vibrant aliveness, or vital lifeforce, of the body that gives rise to an underlying pulse or hum ... This life force arising as a smooth, steady heartbeat ... just as it is. *(Pause.)*

Sankalpa for Your Heartfelt Desire, Calling, or Mission

As you open into the heart space, inquire into your deepest heartfelt calling or mission ... Asking, "If you are a unique expression of life, how does it want to live through you? ..." Abiding as an open curiosity to this heartfelt calling that gives life a sense of meaning and purpose ... A spontaneous desire that you wish to manifest more than anything else during your lifetime ... Perhaps for health, compassion, or awakening ... Affirming and experiencing the felt sense of your heartfelt desire as true in this moment. *(Pause.)*

Sankalpa for Your Inner Resource

Bringing attention to your inner resource ... Resting back and experiencing the felt sense of unchanging Being or feelings of well-being in your body ... A safe haven or refuge that helps you feel secure and at ease ... Welcoming the felt sense of Being and well-being as spacious ... open ... timeless ... perfect ... familiar ... unchanging, yet fresh and always present ... Perhaps a feeling of inner stillness or calm ... If helpful, invite in people or images—a wise person, power animal, object, or place in nature—that nourish feelings of being secure, peaceful, and at ease ... And the felt sense of Being and well-being through-out your body ... Let the images fall away and stay with the felt sense of Being and well-being in the body as sensation ... Know that you can return to this felt sense of the inner resource at any time, day or night, and throughout your practice of iRest ... Whenever you feel the need to feel totally secure and at ease. *(Pause.)*

Rotation of Consciousness with Breath and Energy Awareness

Welcome sensations inside the mouth ... The inner walls of the cheeks ... A pool of sensation in the center of the tongue ... Sense the center of the jaw ... The inside of the ears ... Sense the inner cave of the ear canals, spiraling along the curves to the outer ears ... If there is unnecessary tension ... Sensing right into the center of the tension ... And note what happens ... The skin of the face ... Pure sensation ... The eyes ... sense both eyes as two spheres of sensation resting inside the head ... Feel back behind the eyes to a center point deep inside the head... Feel the forehead... Crown of the head... Back of the head... Sense the whole head as a tingling or vibration... All the while, a deep peace and inner stillness... The ease of Being and well-being. *(Pause.)*

Note the breath just inside the nostrils... The caress of each inhalation and each exhalation as pure sensation... Follow that current of an inhalation as it enlivens sensation into the throat... For several breaths, feel this sensation enlivening the throat. *(Pause.)*

Following each exhalation as a current streaming through the shoulders... The hollows of the elbows... The palms and fingertips... With each inhalation, stay with sensation as it reveals itself... Letting go of memory... Open into pure sensation, feeling from within the hands, arms, and shoulders themselves.

Riding the next current of exhalation as it enlivens the torso... Expanding on inhalation... Releasing on exhalation... For several breaths, sense the inner walls of the torso front and back... left and right... floor of the torso... ceiling of the torso... At your own rhythm, sensing the whole torso... Radiating inwardly and outwardly in all directions.

Following each stream of exhalation as it enlivens the hips... hollows of the thighs... knees... lower legs... feet and toes... For several breaths sense both legs and feet—one feeling—as vibrant sensation. *(Pause.)*

Sense the legs, torso, arms, and head... Feel the whole body, globally, in all directions... Sensing the left side of the body... right side... front of the body... back of the body... above... and below... The whole body radiating inwardly and outwardly. *(Pause.)*

Welcome everything just as it is... Sensations arising and dissolving... All the while, feeling yourself *as* Being... Secure and at ease... Interweaving an inner resource of Being and well-being throughout the entire body... Resting as Being in which all the changing sensations are unfolding.

Sense all that you are now aware of... How sensation is a movement *in* awareness... Feel back into awareness itself... sensing yourself as spacious, unchanging awareness in which all of the changing sensations are arising and dissolving... Changing sensation, revealing unchanging awareness. *(Pause.)*

Meeting Pain with Awareness of Sensation, Breath, Energy, Emotions, and Cognitions

If it feels right, invite an intense sensation in the body...It might be an area of pain that has been present for some time or there may be an area of sensation that is wanting to be seen, felt, and heard in this moment. *(Pause for 15 seconds.)* As you allow this sensation to be here, peel off the label of "pain" and meet it as pure sensation...Noticing if this sensation has a particular shape or texture. *(Pause for 10–15 seconds.)* Is it sharp...piercing...contracted...or diffuse?...How old does this sensation feel? *(Pause.)*

Welcome any emotions, beliefs, or images that might arise with this intensity of sensation. *(Pause for 15–30 seconds.)* Feeling how these may resonate in the body...Knowing you can interweave the inner resource of Being and well-being at any time. *(Pause.)*

If it's helpful, notice if there is a color or substance, notice if it's like a mist, liquid, or an image that's resonating with the sensation...If not, you might assign a color, or substance, to it...Then, join an inhalation, riding its current of breath as sensation just as it is—all the way into the area of intense sensation. *(Pause.)*

As you're inhaling, assign an opposite or different color or substance to coincide with the inhalation...Allow the inhalation with its assigned color or substance to come right into the center and the intensity of sensation with its distinct color or substance...During the pause at the top of the inhalation let the colors or substance blend...Upon exhalation, safely exhale out this new blended color or substance either down through the soles of the feet or up through the crown of the head in all directions. *(Pause for 10–15 seconds.)* Continue in this manner, noting intense sensation with its particular color or substance...inhaling a new color or substance into the center of the sensation...The colors merge during the pause...and the blended color or substance goes downward or upward through the body and out in all directions. *(Pause 30–60 seconds.)* Sensing and breathing this blend of colors, substances...and notice if there're any emotions, thoughts, or images that might spontaneously bubble up...Welcoming everything just as it is...Knowing you can anchor into the inner resource, this field of Being or well-being that is available...ever present...On the next exhalation, releasing the color either through the crown of the head or feet... flowing out in all directions... Setting the breath free to come back to its own natural rhythm. *(Pause.)*

Sheath of Pure I-Ness

Sense all that you are now aware of... How sensation, emotion, or an image are a movement *in* awareness... Feel back into awareness itself... Sensing yourself as spacious, unchanging awareness in which all the changing sensations are arising and dissolving... Changing sensation revealing unchanging awareness. *(Pause 1 minute.)*

If there is a moment of fusing with a changing sensation, daydream, or image, notice how any changing phenomenon is like a cloud simply drifting through the sky... Feel yourself as vast openness, like the sky itself... A field of Being or unchanging awareness. *(Pause 30–60 seconds.)* Something here that's utterly still. *(Pause 15 seconds.)* Whole... *(Pause 15 seconds.)* Complete, just as it is... Untouched by all that's coming and going. *(Pause 30–60 seconds.)*

Note if there're any movements of expectation or anticipation... If so, can you feel it as a reverberation... and set it free, like sugar dissolving into water, to be absorbed as unchanging Being or awareness. *(Pause 1–2 minutes.)*

Sheath of Joy

As you sense your essential nature... the source of Being and awareness... vast, open... note if there is a sense of equanimity or a touch of joy naturally arising. *(Pause 10–15 seconds.)* Perhaps a sense of happiness or pleasure that might be arising... If it feels right, invite in equanimity, pleasure, joy... As it spontaneously arises, notice how it has a distinguishing mark... a sensation that is felt in the body or in the field of Being... If joy is not present, simply meeting what is most calling attention. *(Pause.)*

If helpful, imagine a loved one... a child playing... or laughing with your best friend... An image or memory that brings a touch of happiness, joy, or delight... Then give up images and become completely absorbed in the feeling of pure joy and happiness throughout the body... Feel it as a warmth, radiating from the heart... and with each exhalation, let it spread through the entire body... A touch of happiness or joy saturating every cell of the body... Sense the heart smiling... Perhaps your lips gently smiling... The whole body saturated with happiness, joy, or equanimity... How it may permeate the space beyond the body... Saturating the space of the room around you. *(Pause.)*

If helpful, interweave your inner resource of unchanging Being into your experience of joy and well-being. *(Pause 15–30 seconds.)*

Perceive how every perception, including joy, is arising *in* awareness... Feel back into awareness itself... sensing yourself as spacious and unchanging awareness in which all these changing perceptions are arising... changing perceptions revealing unchanging awareness. *(Pause.)*

Welcoming Everything, Just as It Is

Reflect back upon the journey you've just taken... Welcome the qualities that are or have been present... Feelings... emotions... thoughts... beliefs... sensations... and unchanging awareness in which everything is arising, unfolding, and dissolving. *(Pause.)*

Heartfelt Desire

All the while, the inner resource... a felt sense of unchanging Being and well-being... opening into the heart space... You might sense once again the heart's deepest calling that brings a sense of aliveness and purpose, to which the whole body says "yes!"... And welcome any intentions that support living this heartfelt calling in daily life. *(Pause.)*

Reawakening and Closing

Imagine yourself going about your day while feeling your inner resource of unchanging Being and well-being... And yourself as unchanging awareness, in which all the changing activities of your life are unfolding... Emotions... thoughts... beliefs... sensations... your personality...

And this indescribable sense of being unchanging awareness... Sensing the paradox of being both spacious and vast as awareness—without border or boundary... All the while being this personality that has location, center, and periphery... Your body, mind, and personality free to be just as they are... Sensing and affirming how in each moment you always know the exact and perfect response to each situation that you encounter in life. *(Pause 15 seconds.)*

Take your time now as you transition into your waking life... Allowing the senses to come back online... Allowing gentle movement to arise naturally throughout the body... Perhaps wiggling toes or fingers... Smaller movements expanding into larger stretching... When it feels right, opening and closing your eyes several times while feeling your inner resource of unchanging Being and well-being... Coming into a comfortable position and returning to your eyes open state of waking consciousness... Alert... awake... Grateful for taking this time for yourself and the practice of iRest... Coming fully back to your eyes open, wide-awake and alert state of consciousness and Being.

Stephanie Lopez, LISW-S, C-IAYT is senior director & senior iRest trainer for the iRest Institute. Stephanie's teachings are informed by over twenty-five years of immersion in the non-dual teachings of Yoga. She bridges Eastern wisdom with Western psychology to support transformation. Stephanie leads retreats and trainings internationally with a focus on living an authentic and awakened life. Visit StephanieLopez.org for more.

Resources

Websites

Stephanie Lopez at http://stephanielopez.org

iRest at irest.org for information

References

Shelly Prosko, "Compassion in Pain Care," in *Yoga and Science in Pain Care: Treating the Person in Pain,* edited by Neil Pearson, Shelly Prosko, and Marlysa Sullivan, 234–256. Philadelphia, PA: Jessica Kingsley Publishers, 2019.

Marlysa Sullivan, "Connection, Meaningful Relationships, and Purpose in Life: Social and Existential Concerns in Pain Care," in *Yoga and Science in Pain Care: Treating the Person in Pain,* edited by Neil Pearson, Shelly Prosko, and Marlysa Sullivan, 257–278. Philadelphia, PA: Jessica Kingsley Publishers, 2019.

SIX

Fifteen Minutes for Yoga Nidra

USE THE MEDITATIONS IN this chapter when time is short. They effectively go through all the stages for a full experience, but in an abbreviated manner.

Yoga Nidra 1, 2, 3—Julie Lusk

This starts with tensing and releasing physically using progressive muscle relaxation (PMR) to the count of three. Counting the breath follows for focusing and centering. Unnecessary physical, mental, and emotional tensions are swept away with an imaginary broom to clear the space for insights and creativity to flourish. Time is given for sensing one's experience, just as it is.

Drop Into Yoga Nidra Quickly—Julie Lusk

Lifting and dropping portions of the body is practiced for relaxation, a good substitute for anyone with contraindications for tensing muscles (PMR). A waterway is imagined and used to rinse away tension. Intuition comes alive when an imagined animal appears to give and receive messages. Peace and joy are sprinkled down for absorption.

Into Awareness Now—Julie Lusk

Mindfulness of sounds and using inner vision (chidakasha) clear awareness of distractions. Peaceful contentment, intuitive understanding, and unconditional joy are awakened through guided imagination. Appropriate for practicing inside or out.

Yoga Nidra R & R 2.33—Cultivate the Positive (Pratipaksha Bhavana) —Julie Lusk

Computer lingo and techniques such as scanning, cutting, and pasting are used to apply Patanjali's Yoga Sutra 2.33 which says that when we're disturbed by negative thoughts and feelings, to cultivate the positive.[27] Palming is used to soothe eye strain. There are imaginary links to programs for downloading answers, peacefulness, and more.

27. Julie Lusk, *Yoga Nidra for Complete Relaxation & Stress Relief* (Oakland, CA: New Harbinger Publications, 2015), 186.

Yoga Nidra 1, 2, 3

Julie Lusk

Time: 15 minutes

Summary: This process is as easy to remember as one, two, three. It begins with tensing and releasing physically to the count of three. Counting the breath follows for focusing and centering. Unnecessary physical, mental, and emotional tension is swept away with an imaginary broom to clear the space for insights and creativity to flourish. Time is given for sensing one's experience, just as it is. As usual, a heartfelt pledge (sankalpa) is used at the beginning and the end.

Stages	Process / Techniques
Preparation and settling in	Savasana
Sankalpa	Heartfelt pledge
Physical: Anna-maya kosha	Progressive muscle relaxation to the count of three
Energetic: Prana-maya kosha	Breath counting
Mental: Mano-maya kosha	Sweeping tension away with guided imagination
Intuitive: Vijnana-maya kosha	Experiencing intuition
Bliss: Ananda-maya kosha	Joyful rest
True Self: Atman	True nature awareness
Sankalpa	Heartfelt pledge
Reawakening and closing	

Preparation and Settling In

Feel free to stretch however you like... Settle yourself in as comfortably as possible. It's best to have your head, neck, and backbone aligned. Have your arms beside you with your palms up. Keep your legs and feet straight out, uncrossed, and a comfortable distance apart. You may put a prop under your knees or thighs or simply have your feet on the floor with your knees up. Have your eyes half open or closed. Make some personal adjustments for maximum comfort... Take a nice breath in and sigh it out. *(Pause.)*

Heartfelt Pledge

You're welcome to remember your heartfelt pledge. If you have one, sincerely repeat it three or so times, remembering to be consistent, positive, concise, and as if it's happening right now. Or perhaps let something arise from within you, a quality that supports your highest good and life direction... It's okay if nothing seems to be happening. Trust that it will when the time is right. Or for now, you can use something like, "I am content, more and more," or "My true nature is peace." If this doesn't appeal to you, just skip it.

Progressive Muscle Relaxation

Scan your body mentally, noticing places that are holding tension... places that are feeling relaxed... places that are numb or neutral... Take a big breath in and sigh it out. *(Pause.)*

Tense your right leg muscles. Hold 1 ... 2 ... 3 ...
Completely release 3 ... 2 ... 1 ...
Tense your left leg muscles. Hold 1 ... 2 ... 3 ...
Completely release 3 ... 2 ... 1 ...
Tense your right arm muscles. Hold 1 ... 2 ... 3 ...
Completely release 3 ... 2 ... 1 ...
Tense your left arm muscles. Hold 1 ... 2 ... 3 ...
Completely release 3 ... 2 ... 1 ...
Tense all sides of your torso. Hold 1 ... 2 ... 3 ...
Completely release 3 ... 2 ... 1 ...
Scrunch your eyes and mouth. Hold 1 ... 2 ... 3 ...
Completely release 3 ... 2 ... 1 ...
Tense all over. Hold 1 ... 2 ... 3 ...

Release to relax 3 … 2 … 1 …

You can now release and relax even more to the count of three … 3 releasing … 2 letting go … 1 relaxing even more …

Mentally scan your body, noticing places that are holding tension … places that are feeling relaxed … places that are feeling numb or neutral … Take a big breath in and sigh it out. *(Pause.)*

Breath Counting

Please move your attention to your breath …

Breathe in 1 … 2 … 3 … Breathe out 3 … 2 … 1 …

Breathe in 1 … 2 … 3 … Breathe out 3 … 2 … 1 …

Breathe in 1 … 2 … 3 … Breathe out 3 … 2 … 1 …

Continue breathing this way to the count of three. Each time your mind wanders, simply bring your attention back to breathing. *(Pause about 1 minute.)* Allow your breathing to become effortless and natural.

Sweeping Tension Away with Guided Imagination

You can start using your imagination to sweep away more tension. Imagine having a broom that can sweep and brush away anything that's no longer needed.

To brush away aches and pains, start brushing down your body from the top of your head to your feet, using a sweeping feeling, cleaning out remaining tension and pressure. Do this three or so times. *(Pause.)*

To brush away feelings and outdated emotions, start brushing all the way down your body, using a sweeping feeling. Do this three or so times. *(Pause.)*

To brush away worries and outdated thoughts, brush all the way down your body, using a sweeping feeling, cleaning and clearing away thoughts to expand awareness. Do this three or so times. *(Pause.)*

Continue brushing and sweeping this way as long as you please. Each time your mind wanders, brush that away too and continue brushing and sweeping away what's no longer needed, known and unknown. *(Pause.)*

Experiencing Intuition

Perhaps noticing some clear and empty space opening up … It's free and clear … There's room for insights and creativity to flourish … *(Pause 1 minute or more.)*

Joyful Rest

It's time to notice what's happening and how you're feeling. Perhaps there's a sense of inner peace and joy... If it helps, remember a time when you were happy, or even pretend how it might feel to be happier. Bring it alive by imagining where you were... imagining how it looks... how it sounds... how it smells... enjoying a concept of a happy time and reliving it... Embellishing it to bring it alive mentally, physically, and how it felt... and letting that happy feeling be felt again right now. *(Pause 1 minute or more.)*

True Nature Awareness

You're invited to let all that go and to welcome everything, just as it is, during this silent pause. *(Pause 1 minute or more.)*

Heartfelt Pledge

And from this experience of welcoming and being with everything, just as it is, once more welcome in your heartfelt pledge, your sankalpa. Say it with all your heart a few times. *(Pause.)* Imagine it as true and happening now... Take a big breath in, and let it all go... Trusting that this, or something better, is already unfolding on your behalf.

Reawakening and Closing

It's time for transitioning back, bringing back with you the benefits of Yoga Nidra for yourself and others... As I count from three to one, you will easily and completely awaken. Three, stretching and awakening your body... Two, becoming aware and alert... One, completely wide-awake...

Come up to sitting... Take a few minutes to absorb your experience, knowing there's a place inside that's always there to fully support you on your life path.

Peace, peace, peace. (Om shanti, shanti, shanti.)

Drop Into Yoga Nidra Quickly

Julie Lusk

Time: 15 minutes

Summary: Lifting and dropping portions of the body into relaxation is practiced. This is a good substitute for tensing muscles, as in progressive muscle relaxation, for anyone with cardiac disease, hypertension, glaucoma, or other contraindications. This technique of dropping is carried throughout the Yoga Nidra experience.

Stages	Process / Techniques
Preparation and settling in	Savasana
Sankalpa	Heartfelt pledge
Physical: Anna-maya kosha	Lifting and dropping portions of the body
Energetic: Prana-maya kosha	Progressive breath awareness
Mental: Mano-maya kosha	Guided imagination of a waterway
Intuitive: Vijnana-maya kosha	Experiencing intuition with guided imagination by visualizing an animal
Bliss: Ananda-maya kosha	Joyful awareness
True Self: Atman	True nature awareness
Sankalpa	Heartfelt pledge
Reawakening and closing	

Preparation and Settling In

Feel free to stretch any way you want … Settle yourself in very comfortably. It's best to have your head, neck, and backbone in line. Have your arms beside you. Keep your legs and feet straight out, uncrossed, and a comfortable distance apart. You may put a prop under your knees or thighs or simply have your feet on the floor with your knees up. Have your eyes half open or closed. Go ahead and adjust yourself for maximum comfort. *(Pause.)* Take a nice breath in and sigh it out. *(Pause.)*

Heartfelt Pledge

You're welcome to remember your heartfelt pledge. If you have one, sincerely repeat it three or so times, remembering to be consistent, positive, concise, and as if it's happening right now. Or perhaps let something arise from within you, a quality that supports your highest good and life direction … It's okay if nothing seems to be happening. Trust that it will when the time is right. Or for now, you can use something like, "I have acceptance," or "More and more, I am courageous." If this doesn't appeal to you, just drop it.

Lifting and Dropping Portions of the Body

Mentally scan your body, noticing places that are holding tension … places that are feeling relaxed … places that are numb or neutral … Take a big breath in and sigh it out. *(Pause.)*

- Lift your right leg up a few inches. Hold … Hold … Hold … All at once, drop it back down.
- Lift your left leg up a few inches. Hold … Hold … Hold … All at once, drop it back down.
- Lift your right arm up a few inches. Hold … Hold … Hold … And drop it back down.
- Lift your left arm up a few inches. Hold … Hold … Hold … And drop it back down.
- Lift your fanny up. Hold … Hold … Hold … And drop it back down.
- Lift your shoulder blades up. Hold … Hold … Hold … And drop them back down.

- Open your mouth. Hold... Hold... Hold... And let it close.
- Open your eyes wide. Hold... Hold... Hold... And let them close.

Relax and drop deeper into relaxation even more at the count of three. One, letting go... Two, still more... Three, releasing still further... Feeling the heaviness all over as your body drops into the support beneath you... Sinking down into relaxation even more.

Mentally scan your body, noticing places that're holding tension... places that are feeling relaxed... places that are numb or neutral... Take a big breath in and sigh it out. *(Pause.)*

Progressive Breath Awareness

With your attention on your breathing... sensing your breath coming and going, just as it is. There's no need to change it or fix it, simply breathing just as you are. *(Pause.)*

- Sensing the airflow in your nostrils for a few breaths...
- Dropping the breath down, deep into the chest for a few breaths...
- Dropping the breath down, deeper into the belly for a few breaths...
- Each new breath dropping down to fill up the bottom, filling the middle, and filling the top... and exhaling completely. Continue breathing deeply for several rounds of breath. *(Pause.)*
- Breathing effortlessly now, maybe it's a little slower and deeper.

Guided Imagination

If you like, start imagining a waterway. Imagining what it's like... Perhaps picturing it or getting a concept of it... Noticing if it's calm or rough, running fast or frozen, or something else... Noticing how the water sounds. Perhaps it sounds like a trickle or running smoothly or gushing... Feeling the atmosphere in the air. Perhaps it's damp or dry or crisp... Letting yourself become immersed and mesmerized by the waterway... As distractions arise, feel free to toss them into the waterway to be washed away. *(Pause 1 minute or more.)*

Experiencing Intuition with Guided Imagination

Something catches your attention. It seems to be an animal. And you notice that it's trying to get your attention... What is it?... What's the animal like?... And now it's coming closer ... and you're feeling glad ... and sure enough, you just know that it has a message or perhaps a gift, just for you ... and that's what happens, you are given a personal gift or message from this special animal. *(Pause 1 minute or more.)* And now, you'd like to give something back in return. *(Pause 1 minute or more.)* On your own, say goodbye, just for now.

Joyful Awareness

It's time to notice what's happening and how you're feeling. Perhaps there's a sense of harmony and joy beaming from your innermost Self ... If it helps, imagine droplets of peace and joy sprinkling down, glimmering and sparkling beads of peace and joy sprinkling down ... and being absorbed into your innermost Self, lightening and brightening and soaking in like a time release capsule that can continue to glow and support you. *(Pause 1 minute or more.)*

True Nature Awareness

You're invited to let all that go and welcome everything, just as it is. *(Pause 1 minute or more.)*

Heartfelt Pledge

And from this experience of allowing everything to be just as it is, once more welcome in your heartfelt pledge, your sankalpa. Say it with all your heart a few times ... Imagine it as true and happening now ... Take a big breath in, and let it all go ... Trusting that this, or something better, is already unfolding on your behalf.

Reawakening and Closing

As your Yoga Nidra practice comes to an end, remember that you can drop into greater awareness anytime ... Begin deepening your breath, allowing it to replenish you for optimal energy ... And starting to stretch and move in ways that feel natural ... Waking up, more and more ... Feeling your body moving and awakening ... Eventually, roll to your side for a bit ... Use your arms to lift yourself up to sitting ... Sit for a few minutes to absorb your experience, knowing there's a place inside that's always there to fully support you on your soul path and life journey.

Peace, peace, peace. (Om shanti, shanti, shanti)

Into Awareness Now

Julie Lusk

Time: 15 minutes

Summary: Feel peaceful contentment and energy come alive with the power of sensory awareness. Feel free to practice this either inside or a safe place outside. You will enjoy using mindful listening and inner gazing (chidakasha). Intuitive understanding and inner joy are developed and nurtured.

Stages	Process / Techniques
Preparation and settling in	Savasana and mindfulness
Sankalpa	Heartfelt pledge
Physical: Anna-maya kosha	Sensory awareness with movements
Energetic: Prana-maya kosha	Sound breathing
Mental: Mano-maya kosha	Inner gazing (chidakasha)
Intuitive: Vijnana-maya kosha	Experiencing intuition
Bliss: Ananda-maya kosha	Experiencing joyfulness
True Self: Atman	True nature awareness
Sankalpa	Heartfelt pledge
Reawakening and closing	

Preparation and Settling In

Feel free to stretch yourself... Settle yourself in as comfortably as possible. Remove your glasses. It's best to have your head, neck, and backbone aligned and with your arms out to your sides. Keep your legs and feet straight out, uncrossed, and a comfortable distance apart. You may put a prop under your knees or thighs or simply have your feet on the floor with your knees up. Have your eyes half open or closed. Go ahead and adjust yourself for maximum comfort. *(Pause.)*

Begin sensing where you are, taking it all in … Sensing all that's above … sensing whatever you are on by feeling where your body presses into it … And all that's below it … And now sensing whatever's out to your sides … and beyond … Sensing the atmosphere in its entirety … Take a big breath in and sigh it out. *(Pause.)*

Heartfelt Pledge

You're welcome to remember your heartfelt pledge. If you have one, sincerely repeat it three or so times, remembering to be consistent, positive, concise, and as if it's happening right now. Or perhaps let a heartfelt pledge arise from within you, a quality that supports your highest good and life direction … It's okay if nothing seems to be happening. Trust that it will when the time is right. Or for now, you can use something like, "I am trusting, more and more," or "My true nature is joyful." If this doesn't appeal to you, just skip it.

Sensory Awareness with Movements

Rub your hands like you're washing them … When they're nice and warm, you can rub your face and shoulders, wherever it feels good. *(Pause.)* Lay your hands down where they're comfortable.

It's time to open your mouth to gently move your jaw all around. Easy does it … Now, let your mouth rest, allowing your teeth to part slightly and the corners of your lips to soften and relax. There's no need for any facial expression, so let any tightness or holding fade away, smooth like satin.

With your eyes open, circle your eyes around by gently looking up and circling your eyes around to the right, bottom, left, and back to the top for three or so times. Notice if there are areas where it is not smooth or round. Slow down there the next time to smooth it out. *(Pause.)* The next time you're looking up, pause, close your eyes and rest for a few breaths. *(Pause.)* When you're ready, open your eyes, gently looking up. Start circling to the left for three or so times. Once again, slow down where it's rough or jerky. *(Pause.)* The next time you're looking up, pause, close your eyes and rest for a few breaths. *(Pause.)*

To enhance hearing awareness, begin noticing the sounds around you... Scanning your attention from distant sounds to those nearby... simply taking in sounds as they appear, change, and disappear... There's no need to name them, or even to prefer one sound over another... letting the sounds come to you. *(Pause 1 minute or more.)*

Sound Breathing

And now, listening to the sound of your own breathing... noticing the air coming and going and how it sounds... Welcoming the sounds that breathing makes... Each time your attention wanders off, gently guide your awareness back to the sounds of breathing... Simply listening with curiosity, openness, and acceptance. Listening without reacting or naming the sounds. *(Pause.)*

Inner Gazing/Chidakasha

Even though your eyes are closed, you can still see. Start focusing your inner vision and watch whatever appears on the inside shade of your eyelids and between the eyebrows. It might appear dark, there may be some color or some shapes. It doesn't really matter what's there—what matters is watching whatever comes and goes... There's no need for making comments about it... Let your eyes rest even more now and become quiet, still watching the inner space... softly and steadily gazing and watching in stillness. *(Pause about 1 minute.)*

Experiencing Intuition

All settled and deeply resting and renewing, yet alert and aware. Please rest your awareness at the forehead. *(Pause.)*

It's time for resting in total awareness, a time for welcoming in fresh perspectives, insights, and new understandings... and being ready to receive inner guidance that can come now or possibly later. *(Pause 1 minute or more.)*

Experiencing Joyfulness

Open your attention up to whatever you're experiencing. Perhaps it's a sense of inner peace, of delight, of deep satisfaction. If it's helpful, use your memory and imagination to experience feelings of peacefulness, a time of contentment, of happiness... Perhaps a time when you laughed so hard you could barely stop... or the feeling of jumping for joy... bringing the feelings back alive... and noticing how these sensations and feelings can be relived now... And, if you like, let the memory fade away, not having to rely on events, things, or anything else for being aware of sensations of contentment, joyfulness, and ease, and being in touch with this constant, unconditional inner joy that is always and already yours. *(Pause 1 minute or more.)*

True Nature Awareness

Let this all go for now, lingering and allowing yourself to be present, with your awareness expanding into feelings of being connected, of belonging, perhaps sensing deep contentment... oneness and wholeness. Resting in pure, limitless awareness. *(Pause 1 minute or more.)*

Heartfelt Pledge

And from this experience of welcoming and being with everything, just as it is, once more welcome in your heartfelt pledge, your sankalpa. Say it with all your heart a few times... Imagine it as true and happening now... Take a big breath in, and let it all go... With trust that this, or something better, is already unfolding on your behalf.

Reawakening and Closing

It's time to transition back. Begin sensing whatever is underneath you and supporting you now... Sensing what's overhead... sensing what's all around... sensing your Presence in this space... sensing your body's breath... Noticing it just as it is... Beginning to deepen your breath, allowing it to replenish you for optimal energy... And starting to stretch and move in ways that feel natural ... Waking up, more and more... Feeling your body moving and awakening... Eventually, roll to your side for a bit... Use your arms to lift yourself up to sitting... Sit for a few minutes to absorb your experience, knowing there's a place inside that's always there to fully support you on your soul path and life journey.

Peace, peace, peace. (Om shanti, shanti, shanti.)

Author's Note: Parts of this were adapted from *Yoga Nidra: Guided Meditations for Relaxation and Renewal,* a recording by Julie Lusk available at the HealthJourneys website: https://www.healthjourneys.com/catalogsearch/result/?q=julie+lusk.

Yoga Nidra R & R 2.33—
Cultivate the Positive (Pratipaksha Bhavana)

Julie Lusk

Time: 15 minutes

Summary: Refresh and restore yourself using Patanjali's Yoga Sutra 2.33, which says in Sanskrit, "Vitarka badhane pratipaksa bhavanam."[28] In English this means "When disturbed by negative thoughts and feelings, cultivate the positive."[29] Computer lingo is used to apply this teaching for debugging and reprograming your system to prevent and repair personal crashes while recharging your battery with rest and relaxation. Palming is used to soothe eye strain. You'll do a self-scan of your entire mindbody system using tools like cutting out distractions and defective coding and pasting in something positive. There are links to programs for downloading answers, peacefulness, and more.

Stages	Process / Techniques
Preparation and settling in	Savasana either sitting or lying down
Sankalpa	Heartfelt pledge
Physical: Anna-maya kosha	Body and mind scan
Energetic: Prana-maya kosha	Measured breathing
Mental: Mano-maya kosha	Cultivate the positive meditation
Intuitive: Vijnana-maya kosha	Experiencing intuition

28. Sri Swami Satchidananda, ed. *The Yoga Sutras of Patanjali* (Yogaville, VA: Integral Yoga Publications, 1990), 127.

29. Lusk, *Yoga Nidra for Complete Relaxation*, 186.

Stages	Process / Techniques
Bliss: Ananda-maya kosha	Joyful rest
True Self: Atman	True nature awareness
Sankalpa	Heartfelt pledge
Reawakening and closing	

Preparation and Settling In

Find a comfortable spot for sitting or lying down. Please rub your hands like you're rubbing some good lotion in...To rest your eyes, gently place your palms over your closed eyes, allowing the warm darkness to soothe your eyes for several breaths...Feel free to stretch however you like...Settle yourself in comfortably. Wherever you are, it's best to have your chin aligned with the center-line of your body for clear communication between your brain and body. Keep your arms, legs, and feet uncrossed. Make personal adjustments for maximum comfort...Take a nice breath in and sigh it out. *(Pause.)*

Heartfelt Pledge

If you have one, you're invited to say your heartfelt pledge (sankalpa) three or so times with sincerity. Or perhaps let a quality that supports your highest good and life direction come up...Or for now, you can use something like, "I am focused, more and more," or "I have gratitude." If this doesn't appeal to you, just delete it.

Body and Mind Scan

Start searching your body system by conducting a thorough scan of your physical body, picking up on whatever's going on. Conducting a search of all the places that feel comfortable...all the places that feel uncomfortable...and all the in between places...In your own way, ask for your body's cooperation and support. *(Pause.)*

Start another scan to search your mental components, including your intellect and thoughts...In your own way, ask for your intellect's cooperation and support. *(Pause.)*

Begin another scan of your emotions, including your feelings and mood ... In your own way, ask for cooperation and support from your emotional components. *(Pause.)*

Now, with cooperation and support, become aware of the component that is always running in the background that impartially and neutrally oversees your body, mind, and feelings. It's awareness itself. *(Pause.)*

Measured Breathing

It's time to monitor your breathing. Without changing it, begin measuring your intake of air. Calculate each inhalation by counting how long it takes to breathe in. Do this for several cycles of breath. *(Pause 1 minute or more.)* Determine the average count for your inhalations ... Continue breathing in for that number and breathe out for that number up to twice as long. So, if you're inhalation is four or five, begin breathing out for five to ten. This will help to debug and clear your system of static and noise. When distractions come up, delete them. Continue breathing this way as long as you please. Each time your focus wanders, simply bring your attention back to breathing. *(Pause about 1 minute.)*

Cultivate the Positive Meditation

Imagine there's a blank screen in front of you. It's a clean, blank page. When words, images, or anything else appears, you can choose whatever you want to do to keep it uncluttered and clean.

- You can delete them, so the screen stays nice and clear.
- If it's a negative thought or feeling, cultivate the positive. For instance, use cutting and pasting to delete the negative and substitute something positive. For instance, replace confusion with clarity, or dissatisfaction with satisfaction. It's up to you.
- Use labels. Name it "planning," or "stressing," or whatever it is and continue monitoring.
- They can be filed for now to decide whether to save them for problem-solving later on, trash them, or store them for a while.
- Cutting and pasting can also be used to handle distractions. Just select the distraction and paste something else in. For instance, you can paste in your own mantra if you have one. Otherwise, you can use a peace

mantra like "I am peaceful," or you might like "Shalom." Another one is "Om shanti." Some like to use a word for God, any name will do.

Continue monitoring the mental screen using whichever techniques you want. Just pick some tools to use during this pause. If you doubt yourself, it's just something else to delete, file, or cut. *(Pause about 1 minute.)*

Experiencing Intuition

An insight program is available. Perhaps you're searching for answers to a question or looking for guidance for a situation. If so, look for a link labeled "Intuition." Click on it and let the download happen, making room for insights, answers, and creativity to open. *(Pause about 1 minute.)*

Joyful Rest

It's time for noticing what's happening and how you're feeling. Perhaps there's a sense of contentment... If it helps, open a file that takes you on vacation to a place of happiness. Imagine what it would look and feel like to be on vacation. Or simply stay with whatever is already running. *(Pause about 1 minute.)*

True Nature Awareness

You're invited to let all that go for welcoming everything, just as it is, during this silent pause. *(Pause about 1 minute.)*

Heartfelt Pledge

And from this experience of welcoming and being with everything, just as it is, once more welcome in your heartfelt pledge. Say it with all your heart a few times. *(Pause.)* Imagine it as true and happening now... Take a big breath in, and let it all go... Trusting that this, or something better, is already evolving on your behalf.

Reawakening and Closing

As your practice closes, remember to continue cultivating the positive by changing one thought or feeling for another. When someone is unkind and behaves badly, or when you are tempted to be critical, you can choose to focus on the positive.

Once again, scan your body. In your own way, feel some gratitude for its cooperation and support... Start scanning your intellect, feeling some gratitude for its cooperation and support... And scanning your emotional component with gratitude for its cooperation and support... And some gratitude for that part of you that constantly watches over your body, mind, and emotions.

To restore your energy, bring back whatever you want to save for your sake and for the sake of others... Begin to breathe more fully... Stretching and moving in ways that feel natural... Awakening, more and more...

If you're lying down, roll to your side for a bit... Use your arms to lift up to sitting... Sit for a few minutes to absorb and save your experience, knowing there's a place inside that's always there to fully support you on your life path.

Peace, peace, peace. (Om shanti, shanti, shanti.)

Conclusion

Now it is up to you. Yoga Nidra and its component parts are ready to serve you well from this day forward. Allow it to reveal its benefits over the years. Let its transformative power amaze you.

Knowing about it is not enough—it only works if you do it. Periodic practice is helpful, but regular practice is the best because it builds on itself. The benefits are cumulative. It is relaxing, healing, and can give you the health, energy, and insight to live a life that is deeply fulfilling.

Yoga Nidra is a gift. Like many things, it is often more fun and motivating to share and practice it with others. Why keep this to yourself? Who do you know who would enjoy and gain from this wonderful way of living life?

May you enjoy your journey. Treat it like a lifelong friend. It will always be there for you, and it will not let you down.

Shanti. Peace. Peace. Peace.

APPENDIX 1

Pratyahara and the Rotation of Consciousness

A COMMON TECHNIQUE FOR pratyahara originates from Tantric Nyasa during which a conscious tour through the body is done mentally that corresponds to the brain's sensory-motor cortex (homunculus), energy centers (chakras), nerve channels (nadis), and junctures (marma points). Nyasa, the adding of a mantra or visualization to each point, is a variation that can be incorporated. The rotation of consciousness can be used on its own.

Mentally and systematically scanning the body based on these components clears and strengthens the brain-body connection, accelerates relaxation, and facilitates healing. During the scan, extra time is given to the areas of the body that have more of the brain's sensory-motor cortex associated with them, as seen in the diagram.

The tempo used during the mental scan allows time for each area to be noticed but not enough time to dwell on it or become distracted or bored. This can redefine our relationship with our body. Instead of that achy knee, it is simply identified as the knee. Ignored areas are noticed and integrated. In addition, energy blocks can be cleared during the scan by the movement and flow of life force (prana). The right and left-brain hemispheres are activated, balanced, and equalized as the scan crosses over from side-to-side during parts of the scan. Both the brain and the body benefit from this integration.

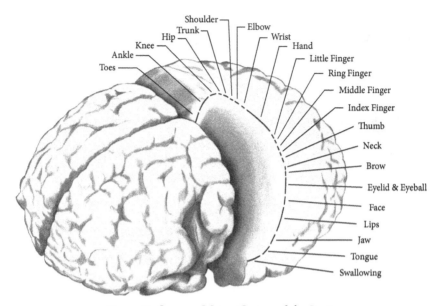

Shoulder — Elbow
Trunk — Wrist
Hip — Hand
Knee —
Ankle — Little Finger
Toes — Ring Finger
Middle Finger
Index Finger
Thumb
Neck
Brow
Eyelid & Eyeball
Face
Lips
Jaw
Tongue
Swallowing

Figure 3: Sensory-Motor Cortex of the Brain

Different sequences are used throughout the book. Some start on the right while others start on the left. Others begin at the head and others at the feet. What matters is that it is effective. Feel free to explore different sequences to discover what you like. Subsequently, consider repeating your favorite sequence from practice to practice by simply substituting it for what is used during the anna-maya kosha state. There are benefits in using the same one most of the time. Not only will it become memorized, the continuity creates a consistent, healthy flow of energy throughout the body and brain.

APPENDIX 2

Chakras: Subtle Energy Centers

CHAKRAS ARE DESCRIBED AS spinning wheels of subtle energy located within one's body that can receive, maintain, transform, and distribute vital energy. Yogis believe they encompass the guiding intelligence of prana, the universal energy of life. They are an important indicator of one's well-being by guiding the developmental stages of our body, mind, and emotions, and awakening our potential as spiritual beings.

References to the chakras are found in ancient and modern Yoga texts. Most schools emphasize seven primary chakras that span from the crown of the head to the base of the spine. Many believe that more chakras are present elsewhere in the body. Each of the primary chakras is associated with and has an influence on physical locations in the body. Furthermore, each is related to stages of psychological growth and human development and has lessons to guide us through life that are integral to our soul's journey. Because they are energetic rather than physical structures, they are not considered as a physical part of our anatomy. Each chakra is associated with colors, an element, symbols, sounds, and more.

Establishing and maintaining balance throughout all the chakras is optimal since one chakra is not especially better than another. Chakra energy currents move both vertically and horizontally, as well as have influence internally and externally. When the chakras are unbalanced with either excessive or deficient energy, the result is physical, mental, emotional, or spiritual difficulties. Fortunately, a wide range of techniques exists to open, clear, activate, and balance the chakras.

Yoga Nidra works with the chakras in direct and indirect ways. Indirectly, this mainly happens through the koshas, especially the prana-maya kosha, and the rotation of consciousness. Sometimes they are focused upon directly as in the Healing Chakra Chorus, the Bihar Yoga Nidra: Intermediate Chakra Visualization, and Welcoming Your Well-Rested Woman meditations.

Here is a list of the names of the chakras going from top to bottom.

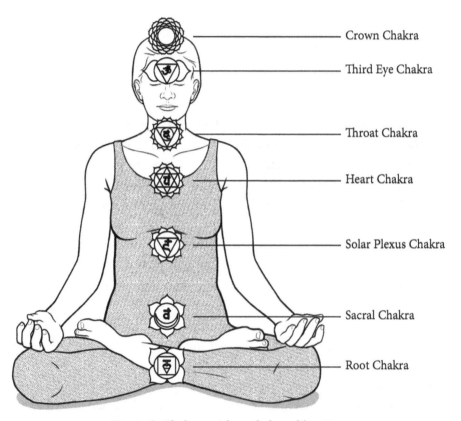

Figure 4: Chakras with symbols and locations

- Crown chakra: Sahasrara (SAH-has-rar-ah) Top of head and above. Associated with wisdom, spirituality, cosmic consciousness.

- Third eye chakra: Ajna (AAHJ-nah) Center of the head, between the eyebrows. Associated with intuition and insight.

- Throat chakra: Vishuddhi (vizh-SHOE-dah) Throat, mouth, ears, hands. Associated with self-expression. Creativity.

- Heart chakra: Anahata (AH-nah-hot-ta) Lungs, heart, arms, hands. Associated with the ability to love and be loved. Forgiveness.

- Solar plexus chakra. Manipura (MAH-nee-poor-ah) Upper abdomen, between the naval and heart. Associated with self-acceptance, self-esteem. Confidence.

- Sacral chakra: Swadhisthana (SVAH-dees-tah-nah) Deep within the lower abdomen and pelvis. Associated with the ability to feel, to want, and to create. Sensuality.

- Root chakra: Muladhara (MOOL-ah-dah-ra) Base of the spine. Pelvic floor, legs and feet. Associated with security and survival.

APPENDIX 3

Yoga Nidra and Brain Wave Fluctuations

PATANJALI WRITES IN YOGA Sutra 1.2 that "Yoga is the restriction of the fluctuations of consciousness."[30] In other words, Yoga *is* the stilling of the movements of the mind, its fluctuations. Yoga Nidra meditation literally changes the "fluctuations of the mind" by consciously slowing actual brain wave frequencies down. It first lowers beta and continues going deeper into the slower frequencies of alpha, theta, and delta as shown below.

Each of us has a brain wave ratio that has a typical and unique pattern. It is composed of percentages of all the brain wave frequencies and is measured in microvolts. This pattern is like our habitual signature. Like handwriting, it usually looks about the same, but it can consciously be changed temporarily to look better or worse. Brain waves vary depending on what we are doing, thinking, and feeling, and whether we are awake or asleep, but the ratios of brain waves usually stay in similar patterns, like a signature. With practice and repetition, these brain wave ratios can eventually be improved. Perhaps our pattern is most often heavy on beta and light on alpha and the other slower brain wave states. Having a high beta pattern lends itself toward tipping into fear and anxiety.

---

30. Georg Feuerstein, *The Yoga-Sutra of Patañjali: A New Translation and Commentary* (Rochester VT: Inner Traditions, 1989), 26.

High levels of beta combined with low levels of alpha deprive us of feeling at ease and make it hard to fall asleep.

Our brain wave ratios and patterns alter our cellular environment in important ways. Depending on the pattern, it can have a positive or negative effect on our physical and mental health. Fortunately, these frequencies can change for the better by consciously using our natural ability to generate different brain wave states of consciousness.[31] When consciousness shifts, it can change the environment in which new cells form for enhancing cell regeneration and repair. As you will see below, different types of cells are affected by a very narrow band of energy and frequencies that are separated by wide ranges of non-effective frequencies.[32] Most of the characteristics and benefits of brain waves on the body-mind were summarized and documented by Dawson Church, Ph.D., the author of *Mind to Matter: The Astonishing Science of How Your Brain Creates Material Reality*.

It is totally possible to retrain the brain, so its pattern has better ratios and becomes our new signature. One that is less stressed, healthier, and more prone to being at peace. For example, alpha waves are the bridge between the conscious, unconscious, and subconscious. If we are rusty on producing alpha, we don't have as much access to the deeper brain wave states and their benefits listed below. Brain waves associated with meditation can shift us into a better place mentally, emotionally, and physically. Church says that feelings of meditative expansiveness are "objective biological facts that can be measured in DNA, neurotransmitters, and brain waves."[33]

Use the info below as a roadmap for how to nurture and experience varying levels of brain waves that occur during Yoga Nidra meditation as we move and fluctuate among its stages. The name of the brain wave as measured in hertz (Hz) is listed first. The ranges given are typically used by most experts. Next, the kosha is noted and the corresponding yogic term for them as identified in

31. Dawson Church, *Mind to Matter: The Astonishing Science of How Your Brain Creates Material Reality* (Carlsbad, CA: Hay House, Inc., 2018), 125.

32. Hans J. H. Geesink and Dirk K. F. Meijer, "Quantum Wave Information of Life Revealed: An Algorithm for Electromagnetic Frequencies that Create Stability of Biological Order, with Implications for Brain Function and Consciousness," *NeuroQuantology* 14, no. 1 (March 2016): 106–125, http://dx.doi.org/10.14704/nq.2016.14.1.911.

33. Church, *Mind to Matter,* 131.

the *Mandukya Upanishad*, a yogic text several thousand years old. Associations describes what you can do to foster those brain wave states and the experience one has based on those brain waves. Next, what is likely to happen during each stage of Yoga Nidra is given. Finally, the benefits and characteristics that can take place based upon the stage of Yoga Nidra and the types of brain waves generated is detailed. Much of this information is based upon associations and is suggestive and not conclusive. More research is needed to further advance this knowledge.

Beta
13–25 Hz

Anna-maya kosha/Physical
Vaishvanara

Brain Wave Associations and Experience
- Waking state.
- Alert. Active. Busy.
- Linear thinking to "monkey mind."

Yoga Nidra Stage
Anna-maya kosha/Physical
- Bodily tension is reduced, which slows beta brain waves considerably.
- Heavy physical feeling.

Focus
- Release of physical tension (anna).
- Increase bodily relaxation.

Benefits and Characteristics
- Normal levels of beta are good for processing information and linear thinking.

- Low beta, from *13–15 Hz* is linked with the body's housekeeping duties.
- High Beta from *15–25 Hz* is associated with fear, anxiety, stress, and the monkey mind.[34]
  - Produces high levels of cortisol and adrenaline and many adverse bodily reactions.
  - Inhibits DNA synthesis, bone growth, and many beneficial cellular functions.
  - Speeds up aging.

Gamma
Subset of Beta
25–100 Hz

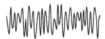

Vaishvanara

Brain Wave Associations and Experience
- Happens while awake or asleep.
- High-level ideas, concentration, learning, and memory processing.
- High IQ.
- Heightened awareness, empathy, and compassion.

Benefits and Characteristics
- Meditation increases gamma.[35]
- Integrates and synchronizes information from all the brain's regions.

34. Church, *Mind to Matter*, 132–134.

35. Antoine Lutz et al., "Long-Term Meditators Self-Induce High-Amplitude Gamma Synchrony During Mental Practice," *Proceedings of National Academy of Science* 101, no. 46 (November 2004): 16369–16373, https://doi.org/10.1073/pnas.0407401101.

- Occurrence of flashes of insight and the ability to perform difficult tasks perfectly.[36]

- Beta-amyloid plaque is decreased by half at *40 Hz*.[37]

- *50 Hz* results in the body increasing its production of stem cells, the "blank cells" that differentiate into muscle, bone, skin, or whatever other specialized cells are required.[38]

- At *60 Hz*, expression of stress genes (cortisol) is regulated.

- *75 Hz* is epigenetic, triggering the genes that produce anti-inflammatory proteins in the body.[39]

Alpha
8–13 Hz
10 Hz is peak

Prana-maya kosha/Energetic
Taijasa

Brain Wave Associations and Experience
- Light sleep. Frequency is between being awake and asleep.

- Sense of being calm and relaxed.

- Presence.

36. Church, *Mind to Matter*, 132.

37. Hannah F. Iaccarino, "Gamma Frequency Entrainment Attenuates Amyloid Load and Modifies Microglia," *Nature* 540, no. 7632 (December 2016): 230–235, https://doi.org/10.1038/nature20587.

38. A. Ardeshirylajimi and M. Soleimani, "Enhanced Growth and Osteogenic Differentiation of Induced Pluripotent Stem Cells by Extremely Low-Frequency Electromagnetic Field," *Cellular and Molecular Biology* 61, no. 1 (March 2015): 36–41, https://doi.org/10.14715/cmb/2015.61.1.6.

39. Laura de Girolamo et al., "Low Frequency Pulsed Electromagnetic Field Affects Proliferation, Tissue-Specific Gene Expression, and Cytokines Release of Human Tendon Cells," *Cell Biochemistry and Biophysics* 66, no. 3 (July 2013): 697–708, https://doi.org/10.1007/s12013-013-9514-y.

- Intuitive awareness.
- State of relaxed alertness and well-being.
- Alpha is turned off by negative emotions, such as fear and anger.

Yoga Nidra Stage

Prana-maya kosha/Energetic

- Dream-like images.
- Thoughts are in the background.
- Sounds like the guiding voice comes and goes.
- Physical heaviness and stillness are felt.

Focus

- Energetic relaxation (prana) emphasizing breathing and chakra balancing.

Benefits and Characteristics

- All brain wave levels of the mind are integrated by alpha, connecting the higher and lower frequencies. Allows consciousness to flow. Tunes the brain to peak performance.[40]
- Neurons in the brain's hippocampus fire at *4–12 Hz.*[41]
- The synapses in the learning and memory circuits of the brain are enhanced at *10 Hz.*[42]
- Synthesis of DNA molecules are significantly increased.[43]
- Improves mood-enhancing neurotransmitters such as serotonin as shown on EEGs.[44]

---

40. Fumoto et al., "Appearance of High-Frequency Alpha Band," 307–317.

41 Church, *Mind to Matter*, 131.

42. Ya-Ping Tang et al., "Genetic Enhancement of Learning and Memory in Mice," *Nature* 401, no. 6748 (September 1999): 63–69, https://doi.org/10.1038/43432.

43. K. Takahashi et al., "Effect of Pulsing Electromagnetic Fields on DNA Synthesis in Mammalian Cells in Culture," *Experientia* 42, no. 2 (1986): 185–186.

44. Xinjun Yu et al., "Activation of the Anterior Prefrontal Cortex and Serotonergic System is Associated with Improvements in Mood and EEG Changes Induced by Zen Meditation Practice in Novices," *International Journal of Psychophysiology* 80, no. 2 (May 2011): 103–111, https://doi.org/10.1016/j.ijpsycho.2011.02.004.

- More alpha activity promotes sound sleep and dreaming.
- Thickens the prefrontal cortex for memory, focus, problem-solving, and emotional stability.
- Facilitates gene expression.
- Improves the immune system.
- Heart coherence (when the interval between heartbeats is regular and constant) is associated with alpha and gamma. It produces an orderly and harmonious synchronization among various systems in the body such as the brain, heart, respiratory system, and blood pressure rhythms.[45]

Theta
4–8 Hz

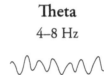

Mano-maya kosha/Mental, emotional, belief systems
Vijnana-maya kosha / Intuition, higher mind, wisdom
Taijasa/Prajna

Brain Wave Associations and Experience
- Light to deep sleep.
- Day and night dreaming.
- Deep meditation.
- Imagery. Flow.
- Intuitiveness. Creative thinking.
- Spiritual experiences.

Yoga Nidra Stages
Mano-maya kosha/Mental, and emotional, beliefs
Vijnana-maya kosha / Intuition, wisdom, and higher mind
- Facilitator is heard in the background.
- Trancelike.

---

45. Dae-Keun Kim, Jyoo-Hi Rhee, and Seung Wan Kang, "Reorganization of the Brain," n.p.

- Perception of colors, shapes.
- Nothingness gap.
- Buoyant.
- Non-attached.

Focus
- Focus is on mindfulness, guided imagery, mantra, etc. (mano).
- Focus is on accessing the higher mind, intuition, wisdom (vijnana).

Benefits and Characteristics
- Free radicals are neutralized by increasing antioxidants.
- Human cartilage cells are regenerated at the *6.4 Hz* frequency.[46]
- Reduction of low back pain can occur between *5–10 Hz.*[47]
- DNA repair is found during theta waves at *7.5–30 Hz.* Antioxidant activity increases.[48]
- Mental and emotional balance occur. Serotonin increases.
- Intuition and creativity increase.
- Consolidation and integration of long-term intellectual and emotional memory.[49]

46. A. Saki et al., "Effects of Pulsing Electromagnetic Fields on Cultured Cartilage Cells," *International Orthopaedics* 15, no. 4 (1991): 341–346, https://doi.org/10.1007/BF00186874.

47. P. B. Lee et al., "Efficacy of Pulsed Electromagnetic Therapy for Chronic Lower Back Pain: A Randomized, Double-Blind, Placebo-Controlled Study," *Journal of International Medical Research* 34, no. 2 (March–April 2006): 160–167, https://doi.org/10.1177/147323000603 400205.

48. E. E. Tekutskaya and M. G. Baryshev, "Studying of Influence of the Low-Frequency Electromagnetic Field on DNA Molecules in Water Solutions," *Odessa Astronomical Publications* 26, no. 2 (2013): 303–304, http://fs.onu.edu.ua/clients/client11/web11/astro/all/OAP_26-2/00 /PDF/56.PDF.

49. Klimesch, "EEG Alpha and Theta Oscillations," 169–195.

- Mindful meditation stimulates functioning of the prefrontal cortex of the brain, promoting memory, concentration, and problem-solving while reducing anxiety and depression.[50]
- Creative flow is enhanced as areas of the prefrontal cortex turn off, decreasing awareness of one's egoic self, self-criticism, and self-control.
- Theta increases in people under hypnosis or in trances.[51]
- Dominant frequency of healers and people in highly creative states.[52]

Delta
0–4 Hz

Ananda-maya kosha/Bliss, unconditional peace, and joy
Prajna

Brain Wave Associations and Experience
- Deep dreamless sleep.
- Meditators, intuitives, and healers are in delta more than normal.
- High delta waves are found in people who are in touch with nonlocal mind, even when wide awake.

Yoga Nidra Stage
Ananda/Joy, bliss
- Yoga Nidra happens when the brain is in delta, yet one remains aware.
- Loss of body awareness. Motionless.

---

50. Yi-Yuan Tang et al., "Short-Term Meditation Induces White Matter Changes in the Anterior Cingulate," *Proceedings of the National Academy of Sciences* 107, no. 35 (2010): 15649–15652, https://doi.org/10.1073/pnas.1011043107; Lazar et al., "Meditation Experience Is Associated with Increased Cortical Thickness," 1893–1897.

51. Carol J. Kershaw and J. William Wade, *Brain Change Therapy: Clinical Interventions for Self-Transformation* (New York: W. W. Norton, 2012), n.p.

52. Robert O. Becker, "The Machine Brain and Properties of the Mind," *Subtle Energies and Energy Medicine* Journal Archives, 1, no. 2 (1990): 79–87, https://journals.sfu.ca/seemj/index.php/seemj/article/view/103.

- Thinking subsides.

- Access to individual and collective unconscious.

- Timeless, spacious sensation.

- Unconditional joy. Blissful.

Focus

- Focus is on being in a sleeping state but with consciousness (ananda).

Benefits and Characteristics

- Profoundly restorative and rejuvenating.

- Consolidates memory and learning.

- Anandamide, the "bliss molecule" is produced, which regulates mental wellness, inhibits the formation of cancer cells, and is associated with feeling happy.

- Neuron regeneration is stimulated at *0.5–3 Hz.*[53]

- Delta frequencies between *0.5–3 Hz* stimulate the regeneration of nerve cells.[54]

- Theta and delta brain waves during sleep clears toxins from the brain. It stops beta-amyloid production, the sticky plaques between neurons in the brain characteristic of Alzheimer's disease, with the greatest effect during delta.[55]

- Growth hormone (GH) secretion is at its highest when delta waves peak in the brain.[56] GH repairs and regenerates cells. This is associated with

53. Betty F. Sisken et al., "Influence of Static Magnetic Fields on Nerve Regeneration In Vitro," *Environmentalist* 27, no. 4 (July 2007): 477–481, https://link.springer.com/article/10.1007/s10669-007-9117-5.

54. Sisken et al., "Influence of Static Magnetic Fields," 477–481.

55. Jae-Eun Kang et al., "Amyloid-b Dynamics Are Regulated by Orexin and the Sleep-Wake Cycle," *Science* 326, no. 5955 (November 2009): 1005–1007, https://dx.doi.org/10.1126%2Fscience.1180962.

56. C. Gronifier et al., "A Quantitative Evaluation of the Relationships Between Growth Hormone Secretion and Delta Wave Electroencephalographic Activity During Normal Sleep and After Enrichment of Delta Waves," *Sleep* 19, no. 10 (January 1996): 817–824, https://doi.org/10.1093/sleep/19.10.817.

the immune system, bone mineralization, muscle mass, fat breakdown, metabolism, protein synthesis, and growth, regeneration, and homeostasis of all internal organs and homeostasis.

- A very low delta band of *0.16 Hz* was found in hippocampus brain slices suggesting that memory and learning may be enhanced by delta activity due to increased activity in the synaptic connections between hippocampal neurons.[57]

- The ends of chromosomes have stretches of DNA called telomeres that protect genetic data, cause cells to divide, and affect aging. Telomeres normally shorten each time cells divide. Meditation preserves and increases telomere length.[58]

- Telomerase, an enzyme that adds DNA molecules to the end of telomeres, shows resonant peaks clustered around a frequency window of *0.19 Hz* and *0.37 Hz* for 10 telomere sequences. Other frequencies did not affect telomerase.[59]

- Delta waves are seen on EEGs when people are having a sense of connection with the infinite.[60]

Turiya
Subset of Delta
No waves
Atman

---

57. Zaghloul Ahmed and Andrzej Wieraszko, "The Mechanism of Magnetic Field-Induced Increase of Excitability in Hippocampal Neurons," *Brain Research* 1221 (July 2008): 30–40, https://doi.org/10.1016/j.brainres.2008.05.007.

58. Tonya L. Jacobs et al., "Intensive Meditation Training, Immune Cell Telomerase Activity, and Psychological Mediators," *Psychoneuroendocrinology* 36, no. 5 (2011): 664–681, https://doi.org/10.1016/j.psyneuen.2010.09.010.

59. Irena Cosic, Drasko Cosic, and Katarina Lazar, "Is It Possible to Predict Electromagnetic Resonances in Proteins, DNA and RNA?" *EPJ Nonlinear Biomedical Physics* 3, no. 5 (May 2015): n.p., https://epjnonlinearbiomedphys.springeropen.com/articles/10.1140/epjnbp/s40366-015-0020-6.

60. Church, *Mind to Matter*, 128.

Brain Wave Associations and Experience

- Beyond the mind.

- Self-realization.

- Pure consciousness.

- Spontaneous and miraculous healing can happen.

Yoga Nidra Stage

Atman

In conclusion, the brain waves experienced during Yoga Nidra can have enormous healing capacity and the potential of enhancing overall health and well-being in remarkable ways.

APPENDIX 4

How to Lead Others in Yoga Nidra

WORKING WITH YOGA NIDRA is powerful. It is up to you to use this book responsibly and ethically. These tips will help you lead clients, students, and friends through Yoga Nidra effectively.

Leaders with little or no training in Yoga Nidra can informally use these scripts with emotionally healthy people. Even still, be careful when presenting unfamiliar themes and techniques with others.

If you plan to offer Yoga Nidra in classes, with clients, or on an ongoing basis, you are strongly encouraged to seek out and complete a Yoga Nidra training and certification course. Most are not restricted to Yoga teachers and welcome mental and physical healthcare providers, ministers, and such. Doing so will deepen your knowledge and experience. It will add to your credibility as well. You will meet wonderful people and enjoy yourself.

Getting formal training is especially important if your groups are composed of people who are unwell emotionally or are unstable. Be sure to seek out special training or professional guidance geared toward their specific needs. Most of the guest contributors, myself included, offer training courses and will be happy to educate and guide you. Refer to the resource list at the back of the book. Investigate trainings that you resonate with and serve the kind of people you are interested in working with. Do not select a program based on convenience alone.

Getting Started

First, familiarize yourself by reading through the meditation script and experiencing it yourself personally. Start out reading what is printed using the tips below. The time frames given are good approximations. They will vary depending on your sense of pacing for each meditation or group. Go for effectiveness. Every word was carefully selected to deliver the best experience. Pauses have been indicated throughout the meditations to facilitate the timing for a favorable experience. You will have to gauge these as you go, watching what is happening with participants. This improves with practice. Eventually, you can start changing some of the wording, so it sounds and feels more like you. After you have the sequence and instructions memorized, you can begin delivering it by heart.

Watch your terminology. It may be a turnoff to use Sanskrit and Yoga terms for those not familiar with it. For instance, Robin Carnes, who contributed "A Beginning iRest Yoga Nidra Script for Active Duty Service Members, Veterans, Families, Health Care Providers, and Support Staff," does not use them with the military population.

It is very important for you to stay in your conscious (alert and efficient) mind. Keep your eyes open. Pay careful attention to all participants. You may have to repeat instructions if you notice that people seem confused. It will also help you with your pacing and delivery.

Preparing the Group or Individual

Begin by sharing the tips in the Quick Start Guide in the introduction to get off to a good start. Adjust the amount of information shared based upon the experience of the group members. That being said, an occasional refresher is helpful.

Briefly describe the process and answer questions at the beginning of each guided Yoga Nidra exercise. Welcome questions and provide appropriate answers. Be prepared with an alternative script if needed.

Let participants know that if they become uncomfortable at any time, they may tune out for a while, open their eyes, or change the visualization. Some of the meditation scripts presented in this book feature time to imagine a place of feeling peace and protection in the beginning, setting the foundation of safety right from the start. It is usually referred to as an inner resource or sanctuary.

Participants can also use this on their own at any time during the meditation itself or when the need for feeling more stable, peaceful, or safe is needed, day or night. See the iRest and LifeForce Yoga meditations for examples.

Optimally, guide others through the entire Yoga Nidra experience from start to finish. Do not rush through it just to get it done in the time allowed. Remember, Yoga Nidra is always about experiencing it and not the technique or method. Give ample quiet time. Always remember to bring them back to full wakefulness at the end.

Reassure people that it is normal for them to follow you for a while and then drift off into their own imaginations, hearing your voice droning in the background. They usually tune back in later. This happens as a natural result of the brain wave states that happen during Yoga Nidra as described in appendix 3. In fact, it is a sign that it is working. If they know this in advance, they won't feel as if they are failing by being inattentive. So tell them not to be concerned and to let it happen.

Setting the Right Atmosphere

Ideally, select a room that has a carpeted floor for lying down or comfortable chairs for sitting. Close the door, shut the windows, and draw the blinds to block out interruptions.

If possible, dim the lights to create a relaxing environment. Low lights enhance the ability to relax by blocking out visual distractions. If the lights cannot be controlled to your satisfaction, use a lamp or night-lights.

Adjust the thermostat so that the room temperature is warm and comfortable. Body temperature tends to lower during Yoga Nidra, which can be uncomfortable. If the room is too cool, it will be hard to relax and remain focused. Suggest that people wear a sweater or jacket if they think they may get cold. Covering up with a blanket is another option; however, it could also serve as a subtle cue that it is time to go to sleep.

When distractions occur—a noisy air conditioner, traffic, loud conversations—try raising your voice, using shorter phrases and fewer pauses, or incorporating the sounds into the guided meditation. For example, you might say, "Notice how the humming sounds of the air conditioner relax you more and more." Or "If your mind begins to drift, gently bring it back to the sound of my voice."

Using Your Voice

Speak in a calm, comforting, and steady manner. Let your voice flow. Speak smoothly and somewhat monotonously rather than in a dramatic fashion to avoid influencing someone's experience unnecessarily with an expressive or animated tone of voice. Do not whisper. Using a microphone helps everyone.

Start with your voice at a volume that can be easily heard. As the guided meditation progresses and as the participants' awareness increases, you may begin speaking more softly. As a person relaxes, hearing acuity can increase. Bring your voice up in tone when suggesting tension and bring it down when suggesting relaxation. Near the end of the guided meditation, return to using an easily heard volume to help participants come back to normal wakefulness.

Tell participants to use a hand signal if they cannot hear you. Advise people with hearing difficulties to sit close to you. Another option is to move closer to them.

Pacing Yourself

Begin at a conversational pace and slow down as Yoga Nidra progresses. Give participants time to follow your instructions. If you suggest that they wiggle their toes, watch them do so, then wait for them to stop moving before going on. If you see fidgeting, add in some permission to adjust and settle back in. They should not be hurried since they have tapped into their unconscious mind (slow, rich, imagery) when they are relaxed and engaged in the meditation process.

Practice will help you develop an effective pace and rhythm. Go slowly but not so slowly that you lose people. Likewise, it's easy to go too fast, so take your time. Don't rush. Using a stopwatch or second hand on a watch can help with the pauses. They usually appreciate ample time given.

To help you with your volume and tone, pace, and timing, listen to a recording of yourself leading guided meditations. It is a bonus that you can then listen to it over and over again, reaping the benefits of Yoga Nidra yourself.

Working with Guided Meditations and Visualizations

Everyone is different. Each person will experience guided meditations uniquely. These individual differences should be encouraged. During a guided meditation, some people will imagine vivid scenes, colors, images, or sounds, while others will focus on what they are feeling or experience it as a concept. All these ways of perceiving are effective. Therefore, a combination of sights, sounds, and feelings have been incorporated into the meditations to ensure inclusiveness of various preferences, temperaments, and styles.

With practice, it is possible to expand your participants' range of awareness. By careful selection and use of images you can help deepen their experience and cultivate their awareness in new areas that can enrich their lives. For instance, a person who is most comfortable in the visual area can be encouraged to stretch their awareness and increase their sensitivity to feelings and sounds.

Using Music

Using music to enhance relaxation is not new. It can set the tone and add to the ambiance for Yoga Nidra. History is full of examples of medicine men and women, philosophers, ministers, scientists, and musicians who use music to facilitate healing. In fact, music seems to be an avenue of communication for some people where no other ways appear to exist. In addition to recorded music, consider using live music. Bells, chimes, wooden flutes, and harmoniums work well.

If you use music, it should be cued up and ready to go at the right volume before starting. Adjust the volume so that it does not drown out your voice. On the other hand, music that is too soft may cause listeners to strain to hear it. Nothing ruins the atmosphere more quickly than the leader having to fool around trying to adjust the music.

Tips on Music Selection

Custom select music for individual clients or classes whenever possible. Not everyone responds in a similar fashion to the same music. Don't assume that the type of music you find appealing will be appreciated by others. Have a variety of musical styles available and ask your clients for suggestions.

Select music based upon the mood desired. Sedative music is soothing and produces a contemplative mood. Fast music increases bodily energy and stimulates the emotions. Select music with a slow tempo and low pitch. The higher the pitch or frequency of sound, the more likely it will be irritating.

Choose music that has flowing melodies rather than sounding disjointed and fragmented. Try using sounds from nature like ocean waves. Experiment with New Age music and space music, much of which is appropriate for this work. Classical music may be effective, especially movements that are marked *largo* or *adagio*. Avoid using familiar melodies because of triggering past associations with the tunes or causing them to be distracted by trying to figure out what is playing. On the other hand, it can be quite effective to use recognizable music if it can enhance and support the intended purpose of the experience.

Matching a person's present emotional state with music is a music therapy principle. If you can match the initial state and then gradually begin changing the music, the person's emotional state will change along with the music. If a person is agitated or angry, begin with faster-paced music, then change to slower-paced selections as relaxation deepens.

Copyright Legalities

It is necessary to have the permission of the copyright owner for any music being played publicly. This includes any class, regardless of the setting or venue where it is held. Copyright infringement violations can result in expensive financial penalties and are time consuming. Here are your options to ensure music is safe to play:

- Purchase a license from the three performing rights organizations (PRO). The primary ones in the United States are ASCAP, BMI, and SESAC.
- Play music that is in the public domain. It can be found by doing an online search for royalty free music.
- Subscribe to an app or streaming service, like YogiTunes, that offers music with a license that covers public performances. A personal subscription to streaming services like Pandora is not sufficient and is illegal to play publicly. You must update your subscription to a business account to be covered.
- Use live music. Either perform your own original music or have local musicians do so. To keep it legal, get written permission from them to play their recorded music if they do not belong to a PRO.
- Play no music at all.

Reawakening and Closing

As you reach the end of a meditation, allow time for them to absorb and integrate their experience. It is important to always help participants transition back to the present. Ask them to sense their surroundings after they are sitting up. For example, suggest they start looking for various colors in the room or have them look for the smallest or largest thing they see, as demonstrated in "Tender Time Yoga Nidra." Encourage them to stretch and breathe deeply. Repeat fitting instructions until everyone is alert. Drinking extra water after practicing is recommended to help with awakening, grounding, and enhancing the detoxifying process initiated during Yoga Nidra.

Processing the Experience

You may wish to add to the richness of the guided meditations by asking participants afterward to share their experiences with others. This is facilitated by creating an atmosphere of trust and confidentiality. Ask the group open-ended questions that relate to the theme of the exercise. Since people will respond in a variety of ways, be careful when describing the expectations and benefits of any given script. Be accepting and empathetic toward everyone. Respect everyone's comments and never be judgmental or critical, even if people express negative reactions. Robin Carnes incorporates this into her script, "A Beginning iRest Yoga Nidra Script for Active Duty Service Members, Veterans, Families, Health Care Providers, and Support Staff."

Cautions

Do not force people to participate in anything that may be uncomfortable for them. Give ample permission to only do things that feel safe. Tell them that if something seems threatening, they can use their inner resource or personal sanctuary, as shown in the "iRest" and "LifeForce Yoga" scripts. Other good options include giving them permission to change it to something that feels right, or they can stop the Yoga Nidra process, stretch, and open their eyes. Emphasize to participants that they are in total control and are able to leave their image-filled subconscious mind and return to their alert rational conscious mind at any time they choose.

In another vein, clients may want to explore what feels uncomfortable to them in the safety of the experience. If you are aware of this beforehand, it is effective to allow clients to read a meditation in advance when introducing challenging concepts or themes that could cause stress.

Advise participants that it is not safe to practice meditation or visualization while driving or operating machinery.

Be certain that participants are fully awake and alert after a Yoga Nidra session and before going about their activities. Have them do some stretches and engage their senses afterward, otherwise it could lead to danger. For example, there are stories of people having trouble driving afterward. One person went right through a stop sign after class. Others have gotten lost on their way home. Another was pulled over for driving too slowly.

Physical and Mental Contraindications

Kamini Desai, the contributor of "I AM Yoga Nidra for Health and Healing," recommends using the option of lifting and dropping the muscle groups and limbs for relaxing physical tension instead of tensing and releasing muscles, as in progressive muscle relaxation, in people with cardiac disease, hypertension, glaucoma, or other contraindications. This is demonstrated in her script as well as by Sri Swami Satchidananda, Viviana Collazo, and the "Men's Health" and "Drop into Yoga Nidra" scripts. "Tender Time" uses minimal rather than maximum muscle tension effectively.

Avoid holding the breath to prevent pressure buildup if conditions like glaucoma or untreated hypertension exist. Have them substitute slow and deep breaths.

Be sure to prop people appropriately for their condition. Refer to the information on savasana in chapter two for details.

Sometimes, students say that relaxation causes them tension. Others will not want to close their eyes during Yoga Nidra. This may be due to a condition referred to as "relaxation-induced anxiety." M. Mala Cunningham says, "This type of anxiety occurs in individuals when they are uncomfortable with 'letting go' and allowing an inward focus."[61] In addition to feeling uncomfortable, it will be difficult for them to pay attention to you. Reassure them that this reaction sometimes happens to people. Take it slowly with them. Give them options to keep their eyes open and suggest they can substitute whatever relaxation strategies are helpful for them. Give them permission to stop their experience at any time by opening their eyes or stretching quietly so as not to disturb others. If you see any of this happening, be sure to discretely and confidentially follow up with them to find out more and give them appropriate support.

---

61. M. Mala Cunningham, "Cardiac Yoga Teachers Training Program" (Charlottesville, VA: Cardiac Medical Yoga, n.d.), 101.

Working with the Military Community

Robin Carnes, the co-founder of Warriors at Ease who has trained over one-thousand Yoga teachers to work safely and effectively in military communities, says that when working with veterans or active duty service members (ADSM), it is important to consider that most are perfectly healthy, both mentally and physically. Please do not assume anything about a service member or veteran's mental health. Even those that do have mental health issues often choose not to readily disclose that information.

The military community is in many ways a parallel universe with its own values and culture. Due to naivete about military culture, even a skilled teacher can be unsuccessful with members of our military communities and cause unintentional harm.

Specialized training in military-informed wording and trauma-informed approaches is needed before working with them and when working with folks who have trauma or traumatic brain injury (TBI) in their backgrounds. For training opportunities, refer to those listed with Robin's meditation and at the end of the book.

Robin advises not to focus strongly on welcoming and witnessing emotions, feelings, thoughts, and beliefs unless you are specially trained to work with trauma, emotional catharsis, and abreactions.

Recording the Scripts

You may record the scripts for your own personal, noncommercial, and professional use. You may not copy, sell, or distribute the scripts to others electronically or in written form without the publisher's written permission. Fortunately, many of the meditations presented here are recorded. See the resource list at the end of the book to get started.

Author's Note: How to Lead Others was adapted and reprinted with permission from Julie Lusk's books published by Whole Person Associates, including *Yoga Meditations: Timeless Mind-Body Practices for Awakening,* and both volumes of *30 Scripts for Relaxation, Imagery, and Inner Healing.* Much of this also appears in *Yoga Nidra for Complete Relaxation and Stress Release,* published by New Harbinger Publications.

Glossary and Sanskrit Pronunciation Guide

CONSONANTS ARE GENERALLY PRONOUNCED as in English. However, the following consonants are pronounced with a slight h sound. These consonants are B, C, D, G, J, K, P, and T. For example, the C is pronounced like ch as in church. The sound of T is as a th in hothouse and not as in breath.

Each vowel has a short and a long form. As shown below, a bar over a letter is used for the long vowels and is pronounced twice as long. The pronunciation guide shows how the words sound phonetically. Sanskrit does not have capital letters.

a as in up

ā as in father

i as in give, pin

ī as in easy (held longer)

u as in put

ū as in rule, cool

e as in may

ai as in aisle

o as in go, Yoga

au as in cow

Sanskrit Pronunciation Guide

A

Ananda (Ah-NAN-da) Joy. Bliss.

Apana (ah-PAH-nah) Downward breath and associated with exhalation.

Asana (AH-sah-nah) Posture.

Atma (AHT-mah) True Self, individual.

Atman (AHT-mon) True Self, universal.

B

Bhagavad Gita (BHAG-ah-vad GEE-tah) Yoga wisdom text, the Lord's Song.

Bhava (BHA-va) Yoga of being. Feeling.

Bhavana (BHA-va-nah) Another word for meditation.

C

Chakra/Cakra (CHA-krah as in chocolate) Wheel. Referring in Yoga to subtle energy centers.

Names of the chakras going from the bottom to the top. See appendix 2 for additional information.

Muladhara (MOOL-ah-dah-ra) Root. Base of the spine. Associated with security and survival.

Swadhisthana (SVAH-dees-tah-nah) Sacral. Deep within the lower abdomen and pelvis. Associated with the ability to feel, want. Sensuality.

Manipura (MAH-nee-poor-ah) Solar plexus. Upper abdomen, between the naval and heart. Associated with self-acceptance, self-esteem. Confidence.

Anahata (AH-nah-hot-ta) Lungs, heart, arms, hands. Associated with the ability to love and be loved. Forgiveness.

Vishuddhi (vizh-SHOE-dah) Throat, mouth, ears, hands. Associated with self-expression. Creativity.

Ajna (AAHJ-nah) Third eye. Between the eyebrows/forehead. Associated with intuition and insight.

Sahasrara (SAH-has-rar-ah) Crown. Top of the head and above. Associated with wisdom, spirituality, cosmic consciousness.

Chidakasha (chi-dah-KASH-ah) Closed eyed gazing focusing attention on the inside of the eyelids and the ajna chakra.

D

Dharana (DAH-ra-nah) Concentration. Steadiness of mind.

Dhyana (dee-YAH-nah) Meditation.

E–F–G

Gunas (goo-nahs) Fundamental forces of nature.

    Tamas (taa-moss) Inertia principle.

    Rajas (rah-jaws) Dynamic principle.

    Sattva (SOT-vah) Balanced and true principle.

H

Hari Om (hah-ree OM) Mantra to Purify and remove obstacles. Opens the heart. Awakens prana (natural energy) in the body.

I–J–K

Koshas in their order

    Maya-kosha (MY-ah- KOH-shah) Maya is illusion. Kosha is layer, sheath, covering.

    Anna-maya kosha (AH-nah) Physical layer.

    Prana-maya kosha (PRAH-nah) Energetic layer.

    Mano-maya kosha (MAH-no) Mental, emotional, beliefs.

    Vijnana-maya kosha (vig-YAH-nah) Intuitive, wisdom self.

    Ananda-maya kosha (ah-NAHN-dah) Joy and peace. Bliss.

L–M

Mantra (man-tra) Sacred sounds and syllables used to guard and protect the mind.

Marma/Marman Points (mar-ma) Vital junctures suffused with prana where flesh, arteries, veins, bones, tendons, and joints meet. Associated with freeing up of blockages of thoughts, perceptions, and emotions.

Maya (MY-ah) Illusion.

Mudra (MOO-drah) Seal. Often refers to a hand gesture.

N

Nadis (NAH-deez) Nonphysical nerve channels throughout the body. Three primary ones are:

 Ida (EE-dah) Located to the left of the spine. Activated by exhalation. Associated with receptiveness, intuition, passivity.

 Pingala (pin-GAH-lah) Located to the right of the spine. Activated by inhalation. Associated with activity, logic, objectiveness.

 Sushumna (sah-SHOOM-nah) Located centrally to the spine. Activated by the gap between exhalation and inhalation. Associated with balance of active and passive nature.

Nadi Shodhana (NAH-dee SHOW-dah-nah) Alternate nostril breathing.

Namaste (nah-mah-STAY) Hand gesture of holding the palms of the hands together in front of the heart. Used as a greeting that means "I honor the light in you that shines in all."

Nidra (Nih-drah/Nee-drah) Sleep.

Niyamas (knee-YAH-mahs) Five tenets for personal living and attitudes toward oneself.

 Shaucha (SAH-cha) Cleanliness and purity.

 Santosha/Samtosha (san-TOH-shah) Contentment.

 Tapas (TAH-pahs) Self-discipline.

 Svadhyaya (svahd-YAH-yah) Self-understanding.

 Ishvara-Pranidhana (ISH-var-ah PRAH-nee-DAH-nah) Devotion to the Divine One. "Your will, not mine."

Nyasa (KNEE-ah-sa) Mentally placing of symbols, mantras, sacredness throughout the body.

O

Om/Aum (Om) Universal mantra. Its symbol is ॐ.

Om Namah Shivaya (Om na-MAH she-VI-yah) Mantra that honors the divine within oneself and others. Destroys negativity and replaces with the positive.

Om Tat Sat (om tot sot) Mantra that means universal truth.

P

Patanjali (pah-TAHN-jah-lee) Author of the Yoga Sutras.

Prana (PRAH-nah) Lifeforce. Natural energy.

Pranayama (PRAH-nah-ya-mah) Control of one's energy, primarily with intentional breathing.

Pratipaksha Bhavana (prah-TEE-pak-shah Bhah-van-ah) Cultivate the positive.

Pratyahara (PRAH-tyah-HAH-rah or prat-ya-HAR-ah) Withdrawal of the senses.

Q–R–S

Sankalpa (san-CALL-pah) Samkalpa (som-CALL-pah) Sacred vow. Resolve.

Sanskrit (SAN-skrit) India's classical and liturgical language.

Savasana/Shavasana/Savasan (Shah-VA-sah-nah) Corpse or sponge pose done lying on one's back.

Samadhi (Sah-MAH-dee) Contemplation, absorption.

Sat (Sot, as in father) Truth.

Shanti (SHAN-tee) Peace.

Shakti (Shaak-tee) Universal creative force.

Sutra (Sue-tra) Concise adage. Thread.

Sadhana (SAH-dah-nah) Spiritual practice.

T

Trataka (TRAH-tahk) Gazing softly and steadily with one's eyes.

Turiya (tur-EE-ah) Awareness of existence beyond the body.

U

Ujjayi (oo-JAH-yee) Ocean-sounding breath.

Upanishad (u-PAH-nee-shad) Ancient Yoga wisdom teachings.

V

Vedas (VA-dahs) Ancient collection of Yoga wisdom teachings.

W–X–Y–Z

Yamas (YAH-mahs) Five tenets for living respectfully with others.

Ahimsa (ah-HIM-sah) Reverence for all life.

Satya (SAHT-ya) Truthfulness.

Asteya (ah-STAY-yah) Integrity.

Brahmacharya (BRAH-mah-CHAR-yah) Moderation.

Aparigraha (ah-PAH-ree-GRAH-hah) Nonattachment, lack of self-indulgence.

Yoga (Yo-gah) Union.

Yoga Sūtra (Yo-gah Sue-tra) Ancient Yoga wisdom teachings compiled by Patanjali.

Recommended Resources

Yoga Nidra Books

Brody, Karen. *Daring to Rest: Reclaim Your Power with Yoga Nidra Rest Meditation, A 40-Day Program for Women.* Boulder, Colorado: Sounds True, 2017.

Desai, Kamini. *Yoga Nidra: The Art of Transformational Sleep.* Twin Lakes, WI: Lotus Press, 2017.

Dinsmore-Tuli, Uma. *Nidra Shakti: An Encyclopaedia of Yoga Nidra.* Stroud, UK: Sitaram and Sons, 2021.

Halpern, Marc. *Healing Your Life: Lessons on the Path of Ayurveda.* Twin Lakes, WI: Lotus Press, 2012.

Kress, Rose. *Awakening Your Inner Radiance with LifeForce Yoga: Strategies for Coping with Stress, Depression, Anxiety, & Trauma.* Lebanon, Oregon: Life-Force Yoga, 2019.

Kumar, Kamakhya. *A Handbook of Yoga-Nidra.* New Delhi, India: D.K. Printworld, 2013.

Lusk, Julie. *Yoga Nidra for Complete Relaxation & Stress Relief.* Oakland, CA: New Harbinger Publications, 2015.

Miller, Richard. *Awakening to Your Essential Nature.* San Rafael CA: iRest Institute, 2018.

———. *The iRest Program for Healing PTSD: A Proven-Effective Approach to Using Yoga Nidra Meditation and Deep Relaxation Techniques to Overcome Trauma*. New Harbinger Publications. Oakland, CA., 2015.

———. *iRest Meditation: Restorative Practices for Health, Resiliency, and Well-Being*. Boulder, CO: Sounds True, 2015.

———. *Yoga Nidra: A Meditative Practice for Deep Relaxation and Healing*. Boulder, CO: Sounds True, 2005.

———. "Welcoming All That Is: Nonduality, Yoga Nidra and the Play of Opposites in Psychotherapy." In *The Sacred Mirror: Nondual Wisdom & Psychotherapy*. Edited by John J. Prendergast, Peter Fenner, and Sheila Krystal, n.p. St. Paul: Paragon House, 2003.

Panda, Nursingh Charan. *Yoga-Nidra: Yogic Trance Theory, Practice and Applications*. New Delhi, India: D.K. Printworld (P) Ltd, 2003.

Saraswati, Swami Satyananda. *Yoga Nidra*. Munger, Bihar, India: Yoga Publications Trust, 1998.

Yoga Nidra Audios

Audios of contributors are listed with their meditation.

Lusk, Julie.

———. *Sleep Relief ~ Yoga Nidra*. Milford, OH: Wholesome Resources, 2019.

———. *Yoga Nidra: Guided Meditations for Relaxation & Renewal*. Cleveland, OH: Health Journeys, 2016.

———. *Guided Mindfulness Meditations: Practicing Presence & Finding Peace*. Cleveland, OH: Health Journeys, 2016.

———. *Yoga Nidra Essentials*. Milford, OH: Wholesome Resources, 2015.

———. *Yoga Nidra for Inner Strength and Balance*. Milford, OH: Wholesome Resources, 2015.

———. *Yoga Nidra for Unshakable Peace and Joy*. Milford, OH: Wholesome Resources, 2015.

———. *Yoga Nidra for High-Level Living*. Milford, OH: Wholesome Resources, 2015.

———. *Real Relaxation: Yoga Nidra CD*. Milford, OH: Wholesome Resources, 2009.

———. *Power of Presence CD with Cultivate the Positive*. Milford, OH: Wholesome Resources, 2006.

Yoga Nidra Training

California College of Ayurveda Yoga Nidra Training from Marc Halpern. https://www.ayurvedacollege.com/Ayurveda/upcoming-workshops-dr-marc-halpern.

Daring to Rest Academy from Karen Brody. http://daringtorest.com/academy.

Divine Sleep Yoga Nidra Teacher Training Levels One and Two from Jennifer Reis. https://jenniferreisyoga.com/divine-sleep-yoga-nidra/divine-sleep-yoga-nidra-teacher-training/.

I AM Yoga Nidra Professional Training from Kamini Desai. https://amrityoga.org/upcoming-all/upcoming-yoga-nidra/.

———. Advanced Trainings. https://amrityoga.org/yoga-nidra/.

Integral Yoga and Swami Satchidananda from Yogaville. https://www.yogaville.org/yoga-teacher-trainings-landing/.

iRest Training from Stephanie Lopez, Robin Carnes, and others. https://www.irest.org/events-landing-page.

LifeForce Yoga Nidra Online Course from Rose Kress. https://yogafordepression.com/product/yoga-nidra-sacred-rest/.

Swami Shankardev Saraswati Trainings. www.bigshakti.com.

Total Yoga Nidra with Uma Dinsmore-Tuli. https://www.yoganidranetwork.org/total-yoga-nidra-teacher-and-facilitator-training.

Yoga Nidra Complete: Levels One through Three Training and Certification from Julie Lusk. https://wholesomeresources.com/schedule-2/yoga-nidra-teacher-training/.

Hatha Yoga Practice

Devi, Nischala Joy. *The Healing Path of Yoga: Time-Honored Wisdom and Scientifically Proven Methods that Alleviate Stress, Open Your Heart, and Enrich your Life*. New York: Three Rivers Press, 2000.

———. *The Secret Power of Yoga: A Woman's Guide to the Heart and Spirit of the Yoga Sutras.* New York: Three Rivers Press, 2007.

Folan, Lilias. *Lilias! Yoga Gets Better with Age.* Emmaus, PA: Rodale Press, 2005.

Weintraub, Amy. *Yoga for Depression: A Compassionate Guide to Relieve Suffering Through Yoga.* New York: Broadway Books, 2004.

———. *Yoga Skills for Therapists: Effective Practices for Mood Management.* New York: W. W. Norton, 2012.

———. Lifeforce Yoga Training from Amy Weintraub and Rose Kress https://yogafordepression.com/level-one-certification/.

Yoga Inspiration and Practice

Devi, Nischala Joy. *The Namaste Effect: Expressing Universal Love Through the Chakras.* Angel Fire, NM: Lotus Flower Books, 2019.

Faulds, Danna. *What's True Here: New Poems and Other Writings.* Greenville, VA: Peaceable Kingdom Books, 2019.

———. *Breath of Joy: Poems, Prayers, and Prose.* Greenville, VA: Peaceable Kingdom Books, 2013.

———. *Limitless: New Poems and Other Writings.* Greenville, VA: Peaceable Kingdom Books, 2009.

———. *From Root to Bloom: Yoga Poems and Other Writings.* Greenville, VA: Peaceable Kingdom Books, 2006.

———. *Prayers to the Infinite: New Yoga Poems.* Greenville, VA: Peaceable Kingdom Books, 2004.

———. *One Soul: More Poems from the Heart of Yoga.* Greenville, VA: Peaceable Kingdom Books, 2003.

———. *Go In and In: Poems from the Heart of Yoga.* Greenville, VA: Peaceable Kingdom Books, 2002.

Lusk, Julie. *Yoga Meditations: Timeless Mind-Body Practices for Awakening.* Duluth, MN: Whole Person Associates, 2005.

———. *30 Scripts for Relaxation, Imagery, and Inner Healing. Vol. 1.* 2nd edition. Duluth, MN: Whole Person Associates, 2015.

————. *30 Scripts for Relaxation, Imagery, and Inner Healing. Vol. 2.* 2nd edition. Duluth, MN: Whole Person Associates, 2015.

Yoga Philosophy

Devi, Nischala, Joy. *The Secret Power of Yoga: A Woman's Guide to the Heart and Spirit of the Yoga Sutras.* New York: Three Rivers Press, 2007.

Durgananda, Swami. *The Heart of Meditation: Pathways to a Deeper Experience.* South Fallsburg, NY: SYDA Foundation, 2002.

Easwaran, Eknath. 1987. *The Upanishads.* Tomales, CA: Nilgiri Press, 1987.

Feuerstein, Georg. *The Shambhala Encyclopedia of Yoga.* Boston, MA: Shambhala, 1997.

————, ed. *The Yoga-Sutra of Patañjali: A New Translation and Commentary.* Rochester, VT: Inner Traditions, 1989.

Mascaro, Juan. *The Upanishads.* London, England: Penguin Books. 1965.

Mitchell, Stephen. *Bhagavad Gita: A New Translation.* New York: Harmony Books, 2000.

Muktibodhananda, Swami. *Hatha Yoga Pradipika.* Munger, Bihar, India: Bihar School of Yoga, 1993.

Satchidananda, Sri Swami, ed. *The Yoga Sutras of Patanjali.* Yogaville, VA: Integral Yoga Publications, 1990.

————. *The Living Gita: The Complete Bhagavad Gita: A Commentary for Modern Readers.* 1st Owl Book ed. New York: Henry Holt and Company, 1988.

Shearer, Alistair, trans. *The Yoga Sutras of Patanjali.* New York: Bell Tower, 1982.

Shearer, Alistair, and Peter Russell, trans. *The Upanishads.* New York: Bell Tower, 1978.

Yoga Nidra Research

iRest Yoga Nidra research is located at http://www.irest.us/research.

Kumar, Kamakhya. Research on Yoga Nidra, under the direction of Kamakhya Kumar, PhD., is located at http://yoganidra.webs.com/researchpublication.htm.

Bibliography

Adhana, Ritu, Rani Gupta, Jyoti Dvivedii, and Sohaib Ahmad. "The Influence of the 2:1 Yogic Breathing Technique on Essential Hypertension." *Indian Journal of Physiology and Pharmacology* 57, no. 1 (January-March 2013): 38–44. http://www.ncbi.nlm.nih.gov/pubmed/24020097.

Afonso, Rui Ferreira, Helena Hachul, Elisa Harumi Kozasa, Denise de Souza oliveira, Viviane Goto, Dinah Rodrigues, Sérgio Tufik, and José Robert Leite. "Yoga Decreases Insomnia in Postmenopausal Women: A Randomized Clinical Trial." *Menopause* 19, no. 2 (February 2012):186–193. http://www.ncbi.nlm.nih.gov/pubmed/22048261.

Ahmed, Zaghloul, and Andrzej Wieraszko. "The Mechanism of Magnetic Field-Induced Increase of Excitability in Hippocampal Neurons." *Brain Research* 1221 (July 2008): 30–40. https://doi.org/10.1016/j.brainres.2008.05.007.

Amita, S., S. Prabhakar, I. Manoj, S. Harminder, and T. Pavan. "Effect of Yoga-Nidra on Blood Glucose Level in Diabetic Patients." *Indian Journal of Physiological and Pharmacology* 53, no. 1 (Janury–March 2009): 97–101. https://pubmed.ncbi.nlm.nih.gov/19810584/.

Ardeshirylajimi, A., and M. Soleimani. "Enhanced Growth and Osteogenic Differentiation of Induced Pluripotent Stem Cells by Extremely Low-Frequency Electromagnetic Field." *Cellular and Molecular Biology* 61, no. 1 (March 2015): 36–41. https://pubmed.ncbi.nlm.nih.gov/25817344/.

Becker, Robert O. "The Machine Brain and Properties of the Mind." *Subtle Energies and Energy Medicine Journal Archives* 1, no. 2 (1990): 79–87. https://journals.sfu.ca/seemj/index.php/seemj/article/view/103.

Benson, Herbert, and Richard Friedman. "Harnessing the Power of the Placebo Effect and Renaming It 'Remembered Wellness.'" *Annual Review of Medicine* 47 (February 1996): 193–199. https://www.ncbi.nlm.nih.gov/pubmed/8712773.

Benson, Herbert, and William Proctor. *Relaxation Revolution: Enhancing Your Personal Health Through the Science and Genetics of Mind Body Healing.* New York: Scribner, 2010.

Church, Dawson. *Mind to Matter: The Astonishing Science of How Your Brain Creates Material Reality.* Carlsbad, CA: Hay House., Inc., 2018.

Collazo, Viviana. "Journey Through a Conscious Spiritual Pregnancy and Birthing." PhD diss., Orlando, FL. Alliance of Divine Love Doctorate Program, 2009.

Cosic, Irena, Drasko Cosic, and Katarina Lazar. "Is It Possible to Predict Electromagnetic Resonances in Proteins, DNA and RNA?" *EPJ Nonlinear Biomedical Physics* 3, no. 5 (May 2015): n.p. https://epjnonlinearbiomedphys.springeropen.com/articles/10.1140/epjnbp/s40366-015-0020-6.

Cunningham, M. Mala. "Cardiac Yoga Teachers Training Program." Charlottesville, VA: Cardiac Medical Yoga, n.d.

De Girolamo, Laura, Deborah Stanco, Emanuela Galliera, Marco Viganò, Alessandra Colombini, Stefania Setti, Elena Vianello, Massimiliano Marco Corsi Romanelli, Valerio Sansone. "Low Frequency Pulsed Electromagnetic Field Affects Proliferation, Tissue-Specific Gene Expression, and Cytokines Release of Human Tendon Cells." *Cell Biochemistry and Biophysics* 66, no. 3 (July 2013): 697–708. https://doi.org/10.1007/s12013-013-9514-y.

Desai, Kamini, *Yoga Nidra: The Art of Transformational Sleep.* Twin Lakes, WI: Lotus Press, 2017.

Dias da Silva, V.J. and Paton, J.F.R. (2012), The interplay between the autonomic and immune systems. Experimental Physiology, 97: 1143–1145. doi:10.1113/expphysiol.2011.061473.

Faulds, Danna. *Go In and in: Poems from the Heart of Yoga.* Greenville, VA: Peaceable Kingdom Books, 2002.

Feuerstein, Georg. *The Shambhala Encyclopedia of Yoga.* Boston, MA: Shambhala: 1997.

———. *The Yoga-Sutra of Patañjali: A New Translation and Commentary.* Rochester VT: Inner Traditions, 1989.

Folan, Lilias. *Lilias! Yoga Gets Better with Age.* Emmaus, PA: Rodale Press: 2005.

Fumoto, Masaki, Ikuko Sato-Suzuki, Yoshinari Seki, and Hideho Arita. "Appearance of High-Frequency Alpha Band with Disappearance of Low-Frequency Alpha Band in EEG is Produced During Voluntary Abdominal Breathing In and Eyes-Closed Condition." *Neuroscience Research* 50, no. 3 (November 2004): 307–317. https://doi.org/10.1016/j.neures.2004.08.005.

Fumoto, Masaki, Tsutomu Oshima, Kiyoshi Kamiya, Hiromi Kikuchi, Yoshinari Seki, Yasushi Nakatani, Xinjun Yu, Tamami Sekiyama, Ikuko Sato-Suzuki, Hideho Arita. "Ventral Prefrontal Cortex and Serotonergic System Activation During Pedaling Exercise Induces Negative Mood Improvement and Increased Alpha Band in EEG." *Behavioral Brain Research* 213, no. 1 (November 2010): 1–9. https://doi.org/10.1016/j.bbr.2010.04.017.

Geesink, Hans J. H., and Dirk K. F. Meijer. "Quantum Wave Information of Life Revealed: An Algorithm for Electromagnetic Frequencies that Create Stability of Biological Order, with Implications for Brain Function and Consciousness." *NeuroQuantology* 14, no. 1 (January 2016): http://dx.doi.org/10.14704/nq.2016.14.1.911.

Gothe, Neha, Matthew B. Pontifex, Charles Hillman, and Edward McAuley. "The Acute Effects of Yoga on Executive Function." *Journal of Physical Activity and Health* 10, no. 4 (May 2013): 488–495. https://doi.org/10.1123/jpah.10.4.488.

Gronifier, C., R. Luthringer, M. Follenius, N. Schaltenbrand, J. P. Macher, A. Muzet A, and G. Brandenberger. "A Quantitative Evaluation of the Relationships Between Growth Hormone Secretion and Delta Wave Electroencephalographic Activity During Normal Sleep and After Enrichment in Delta Waves." *Sleep* 19, no. 10 (January 1996): 817–824. https://doi .org/10.1093/sleep/19.10.817.

Grøntved, Anders, An Pan, Rania A. Mekary, Meir Stampfer, Walter C. Willett, JoAnn E. Manson, and Frank B. Hu. "Muscle-Strengthening and Conditioning Activities and Risk of Type 2 Diabetes: A Prospective Study in Two Cohorts of US Women." *PLOS Medicine* 11, no. 1 (January 2014): n.p. https://doi.org/10.1371/journal.pmed.1001587.

Hagelin, John. "Stress Prevention: Its Impact on Health and Medical Savings." *Institute of Science Technology and Public Policy.* Congressional Prevention Coalition, 1998.

Hölzel, Britta, K., James Carmody, Mark Vangel, Christina Congleton, Sita M. Yerramsetti, Tim Gard, and Sara W. Lazar. "Mindfulness Practice Leads to Increases in Regional Brain Gray Matter Density." *Psychiatry Research: Neuroimaging* 191, no. 1 (January 2011): 36–43. https://dx .doi.org/10.1016%2Fj.pscychresns.2010.08.006.

Iaccarino, Hannah F., Annabelle C. Singer, Anthony J. Martorell, Andrii Rudenko, Fan Gao, Tyler Z. Gillingham, Hansruedi Mathys et al. "Gamma Frequency Entrainment Attenuates Amyloid Load and Modifies Microglia." *Nature* 540, no. 7632 (December 2016): 230–235. https://doi .org/10.1038/nature20587.

Jacobs, Tonya L., Elissa S. Epel, Jue Lin, Elizabeth H. Blackburn, Owen M. Wolkowitz, David A. Bridwell, Anthony P. Zanesco, et al. "Intensive Meditation Training, Immune Cell Telomerase Activity, and Psychological Mediators." *Psychoneuroendocrinology* 36, no. 5 (2011): 664–681. https:// doi.org/10.1016/j.psyneuen.2010.09.010.

Kang, Jae-Eun, Miranda M. Lim, Randall J. Bateman, James J. Lee, Liam P. Smyth, John R. Cirrito, Nobuhiro Fujiki, Seiji Nishino, and David M. Holtzman. "Amyloid-b Dynamics Are Regulated by Orexin and the Sleep-Wake Cycle." *Science* 326, no. 5955 (November 2009): 1005–1007. https://dx.doi.org/10.1126%2Fscience.1180962.

Kershaw, Carol J., and J. William Wade. *Brain Change Therapy: Clinical Interventions for Self-Transformation.* New York: W. W. Norton, 2012.

Kiecolt-Glaser, Janice K., Jeanette M. Bennett, Rebecca Andridge, Juan Peng, Charles L. Shapiro, William B. Malarkey, Charles F. Emery, Rachel Layman, Ewa E. Mrozek, and Ronald Glaser. "Yoga's Impact on Inflammation, Mood, and Fatigue in Breast Cancer Survivors: A Randomized Controlled Trial." *Journal of Clinical Oncology* 32, no. 10 (April 2014): 1040–1049. https://dx.doi.org/10.1200%2FJCO.2013.51.8860.

Kim, Dae-Keun, Jyoo-Hi Rhee, Seung Wan Kang. "Reorganization of the Brain and Heart Rhythm During Autogenic Meditation." *Frontiers in Integrative Neuroscience* 7, 109 (2013). https://dx.doi.org/10.3389%2Ffnint .2013.00109.

Klimesch, Wolfgang. "EEG Alpha and Theta Oscillations Reflect Cognitive and Memory Performance: A Review and Analysis." *Brain Research Reviews* 29, no. 2–3 (April 1999): 169–195. https://doi.org/10.1016/S0165 -0173(98)00056-3.

Krishna Bandi Hri, Pravati Pal, Pal G. K., Balachander J., Jayasettiaseelon E., Sreekanth Y., Sridhar M. G., and Guar G., S. "Effect of Yoga Therapy on Heart Rate, Blood Pressure and Cardiac Autonomic Function in Heart Failure." *Journal of Clinical & Diagnostic Research* 8, no. 1 (January 2014):14–16. http://www.ncbi.nlm.nih.gov/pubmed/24596712.

Kumar, Kamakhya. *A Handbook of Yoga-Nidra.* New Delhi, India: D. K. Printworld, 2013.

———. "A Holistic Approach to Stress Management." *Nature & Wealth* 7, no.4 (October 2008): n. p. https://www.researchgate.net/publication /260268320_Holistic_approach_to_Stress_management.

———. "A Study of the Improvement of Physical and Mental Health Through 'Yoga Nidra.'" *Dev Sanskriti Inter-Disciplinary Research Journal* 4, no. 4 (January 2006): 39–46, https://www.researchgate.net/publication/21545 1321_A_study_of_the_improvement_of_Physical_and_Mental_Health _through_Yoga_nidra.

———. "A Study on the Impact on Stress and Anxiety Through Yoga Nidra." *Indian Journal of Traditional Knowledge, NISCAIR, New Delhi* 7, no. 3 (July

2008): 401–404 and 405–409. https://www.researchgate.net
/publication/215448826_A_study_on_the_impact_on_stress_and
_anxiety_through_Yoga_nidra.

———. "Complete the Course of Sleep Through Yoga Nidra." *Nature &
Wealth* 7 no. 1 (Jan 2008): n. p. https://www.researchgate.net
/publication/215461447_Complete_the_Course_of_Sleep_through_Yoga
_Nidra.

———. "Effect of *Yoga Nidra* on Hypertension & Other Psychological Co-relates." *Yoga the Science Journal* 3, no. 7 (2005): n.p. https://www.research
gate.net/profile/Kamakhya_Kumar/publication/215451330_Effect_of
_Yoga_nidra_on_hypertension_other_psychological_co-relates/links/00b4
9529ed404101e6000000/Effect-of-Yoga-nidra-on-hypertension-other
-psychological-co-relates.pdf.

———. "Manage the Psycho-Complexities Through Yoga Nidra." National
Conference on Yoga Therapy, organized at Manglore University, Manglore,
Karnataka, India, 2013. https://www.researchgate.net/publication
/254863532_Manage_the_psycho-complexities_through_Yoga_Nidra.

———. "Origin and Application of Yoga Nidra." *Nature & Wealth* 4 No. 4
(September 2015): n.p.

———. "Psychological Changes as Related to Yoga Nidra." *International Journal of Psychology: A Biopsychosocial Approach* 6 (2010): 129–137. https://
www.researchgate.net/publication/213341724_Psychological_changes
_as_related_to_Yoga_Nidra.

———. "Reversing the Ischemic Heart Disease Through Yogic Relaxation."
National Yoga Week, organized by Morarji Desai National Institute of Yoga,
New Delhi. *Nature and Wealth* 3, no. 1 (January 2009): n. p. https://www
.researchgate.net/publication/215585754_Reversing_the_Ischemic_Heart
_Disease_through_Yoga_Nidra.

———. "Stress Free Life Through Yoga Nidra." International Symposium on
Yogism (December 2010): 36–38. https://www.researchgate.net/publication
/215455731_Stress_Free_Life_through_Yoga_nidra.

———. "The Healing Sleep." *Yoga Magazine (Body Mind Spirit)*. Issue 50,
2007.

———. "Yoga Nidra and Its Impact on Blood Cells." *National Yoga Week*, organized by Morarji Desai National Institute of Yoga, New Delhi (2007): n. p.

———. "*Yoga Nidra* and Its Impact on Student's Wellbeing." *Yoga Mimamsa* 36, no. 1 (April 2004): 31–35. https://www.researchgate.net/publication /215451327_Yoga_nidra_and_its_impact_on_student%27s_well_being.

Kumar, Kamakhya, and Bhanu Joshi. "Study on the Effect of *Pranakarshan Pranayama* & *Yoga Nidra* on Alpha EEG & GSR." *Indian Journal of Traditional Knowledge* 8, no. 3 (July 2009): 453–454. https://www.researchgate .net/publication/201888482_Study_on_the_Effect_of_Yoga_Nidra _Pranakarshan_Pranayama_on_Alpha_EEG_GSR.

Kumar, Kamakhya, and Pranav Pandya. "A Study on the Impact on ESR Level Through Yogic Relaxation Technique *Yoga Nidra*." *Indian Journal of Traditional Knowledge* 11, no. 2 (April 2012): 358–361. http://nopr.niscair.res.in /bitstream/123456789/13871/1/IJTK%2011%282%29%20358–361.pdf.

Lazar, Sara W., Catherine E. Kerr, Rachel H. Wasserman, Jeremy R. Gray, Douglas N. Greve, Michael T. Treadway, Metta McGarvey et al. "Meditation Experience Is Associated with Increased Cortical Thickness." *Neuroreport* 16, no. 17 (November 2005): 1893–1897. https://doi.org/10.1097/01 .wnr.0000186598.66243.19.

Lee, P. B., Y. C. Kim, Y. J. Lim, C. J. Lee, S. S. Choi, S. H. Park, J. G. Lee, S. C. Lee. "Efficacy of Pulsed Electromagnetic Therapy for Chronic Lower Back Pain: A Randomized, Double-Blind, Placebo-Controlled Study." *Journal of International Medical Research* 34 no. 2 (March–April 2006): 160–167. https://doi.org/10.1177/147323000603400205.

Lusk, Julie. *Yoga Nidra for Complete Relaxation & Stress Relief.* Oakland, CA: New Harbinger Publications, 2015.

Lutz, Antoine, Lawrence L. Grieschar, Nancy B. Rawlings, Matthieu Ricard, and Richard J. Davidson. "Long-Term Mediators Self-Induce High-Amplitude Gamma Synchrony During Mental Practice." *Proceedings of the National Academy of Sciences* 101, no. 46 (November 2004): 1639–16373. https://doi.org/10.1073/pnas.0407401101.

Mankar, Sumedh. "Effects of Utilizing Yoga Nidra on Reducing Symptoms of Depression and Anxiety in a Psychiatric Population." *The Journal of the American Osteopathic Association* 112 no. 8 (2012): 543. Abstract C19.

McGonigal, Kelly. "Inspired Intention: The Nature of Sankalpa." *Yoga International* (Winter 2010–2011): 44–49.

Panda, Nursingh Charan. *Yoga-Nidra: Yogic Trance Theory, Practice and Applications.* New Delhi, India: D.K. Printworld (P) Ltd., 2003.

Pandya, P., and Kamakhya Kumar. "Yoga Nidra and Its Impact on Human Physiology." *Yoga Vijnan, MDNIY,* New Delhi 1 no. 1, (January 2008): 1–8. https://www.researchgate.net/publication/260268130_Yoga_Nidra _Its_impact_on_Human_Physiology.

Prosko, Shelly. "Compassion in Pain Care." In *Yoga and Science in Pain Care: Treating the Person in Pain*, edited by Neil Pearson, Shelly Prosko, and Marlysa Sullivan, 234–256. Philadelphia, PA: Jessica Kingsley Publishers, 2019.

Rani, Khushbu, Sc Tiwari, Uma Singh, Gg Agrawal, Archana Ghildiyal, and Neena Srivastava. 2011. "Impact of Yoga Nidra on Psychological General Wellbeing in Patients with Menstrual Irregularities: A Randomized Controlled Trial." *International Journal of Yoga* 4, no. 1 (January 2011): 20–25. https://doi.org/10.4103/0973-6131.78176.

Saki, A., K. Suzuki, T. Nakamura, T. Norimura, T. Tsuchiya. "Effects of Pulsing Electromagnetic Fields on Cultured Cartilage Cells." *International Orthopaedics* 15, no. 4 (1991): 341–346. https://doi.org/10.1007 /bf00186874.

Satchidananda, Sri Swami, ed. *The Yoga Sutras of Patanjali.* Yogaville, VA: Integral Yoga Publications, 1990.

Sivananda, Swami. Sivananda Online. "Pratyahara." Accessed June 29, 2020. http://www.sivanandaonline.org/public_html/?cmd=displaysection& section_id=893.

Sisken, Betty F., Paul Midkiff, Andrew Tweheus, and Marko Markov. "Influence of Static Magnetic Fields on Nerve Regeneration In Vitro." *Environmentalist* 27, no. 4 (2007): 477–481. https://link.springer.com/article /10.1007/s10669-007-9117-5.

Sodhi, Candy, Sheena Singh, and Amit Bery. "Assessment of the Quality of Life in Patients with Bronchial Asthma, Before and After Yoga: A Randomised Trial." *Iranian Journal of Allergy, Asthma, and Immunology* 13, no. 1 (February 2014): 55–60. http://www.ncbi.nlm.nih.gov/pubmed/24338229.

Stetter, Friedhelm, Sirko Kupper. "Autogenic Training: A Meta-Analysis of Clinical Outcome Studies." *Applied Psychophysiology and Biofeedback* 27, no 1 (March 2002): 45–98. https://doi.org/10.1023/a:1014576505223.

Sullivan, Marlysa. "Connection, Meaningful Relationship, and Purpose in Life: Social and Existential Concerns in Pain Care." In *Yoga and Science in Pain Care: Treating the Person in Pain*, edited by Neil Pearson, Shelly Prosko, and Marlysa Sullivan, 257–278. Philadelphia, PA: Jessica Kingsley Publishers, 2019.

Takahashi, K., I. Kaneko, M. Date, and E. Fukada, E. "Effect of Pulsing Electromagnetic Fields on DNA Synthesis in Mammalian Cells in Culture." *Experientia* 42, no. 2 (February 1986): 185–186. https://doi.org/10.1007/bf01952459.

Tang, Ya-Ping, Eiji Shimizu, Gilles Dube, Claire Rampon, Geoffrey A. Kerchner, Min Zhuo, Guosong Liu, and Joe Z. Tsien. "Genetic Enhancement of Learning and Memory in Mice." *Nature* 401, no. 6748 (September 1999): 63–69. https://doi.org/10.1038/43432.

Tang, Yi-Yuan, Qilin Lu, Xiujuan Geng, Elliot A. Stein, Yihong Yang, and Michael I. Posner. "Short-Term Meditation Induces White Matter Changes in the Anterior Cingulate." *Proceedings of the National Academy of Sciences* 107, no. 35 (August 2010): 15649–15652. https://doi.org/10.1073/pnas.1011043107.

Tekutskaya, E. E., and M. G. Baryshev. "Studying of Influence of the Low-Frequency Electromagnetic Field on DNA Molecules in Water Solutions." *Odessa Astronomical Publications* 26, no. 2 (2013): 303–304. http://fs.onu.edu.ua/clients/client11/web11/astro/all/OAP_26-2/00/PDF/56.PDF.

Turner, Toko-pa. *Belonging: Remembering Ourselves Home.* Salt Spring Island, British Columbia: Her Own Room Press, 2017.

Waltke, Bruce K. "Heart." Bible Study Tools. Salem Media Group. Accessed October 21, 2020. https://www.biblestudytools.com/dictionary/heart/.

Yu, Xinjun, Masaki Fumoto, Yasushi Nakatani, Tamami Sekiyama, Hiromi Kikuchi, Yoshinari Seki, Ikuko Sato-Suzuki, Hideho Arita. "Activation of the Anterior Prefrontal Cortex and Serotonergic System Is Associated with Improvements in Mood and EEG Changes Induced by Zen Meditation Practice in Novices." *International Journal of Psychophysiology* 80, no. 2 (May 2011): 103–111. https://doi.org/10.1016/j.ijpsycho.2011.02.004.

Credits

Trademarked Material

These credits were provided by the author. Additional trademarks may apply to the materials owned by the individual contributors.

Jennifer Reis: Divine Sleep® and Five Element Yoga®

Sri Swami Satchidananda: Integral Yoga®

Mala Cunningham: Cardiac Yoga®

Kamini Desai: I AM Yoga Nidra™

Rose Kress and Amy Weintraub: LifeForce Yoga™

Marc Halpern: Yoga Nidra and Self-Healing™ ©

Karen Brody: Daring to Rest™ ©

iRest®

Additional Credits and Permissions

Author photo credit: Stuart McClay Smith

Atman Kosha Labyrinth illustration design on page 16 is by the author.